MW01026762

Radiation Safety in Nuclear Medicine

Second Edition

Radiation Safety in Nuclear Medicine

Second Edition

Max H. Lombardi

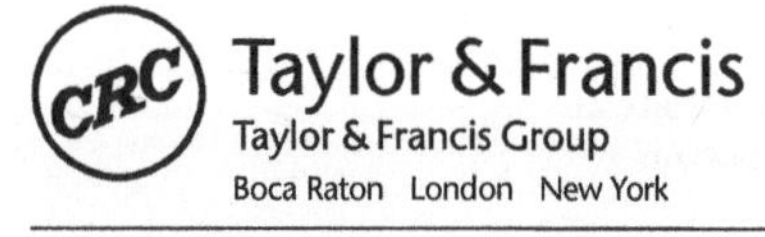

CRC is an imprint of the Taylor & Francis Group,
an informa business

CRC Press
Taylor & Francis Group
6000 Broken Sound Parkway NW, Suite 300
Boca Raton, FL 33487-2742

Printed in the United States of America on acid-free paper
10 9 8 7 6 5 4 3 2 1

International Standard Book Number-10: 0-8493-8168-1 (Hardcover)
International Standard Book Number-13: 978-0-8493-8168-3 (Hardcover)

Library of Congress Cataloging-in-Publication Data

Lombardi, Max H., 1932-
Radiation safety in nuclear medicine / Max H. Lombardi. -- 2nd ed.
p. cm.
Includes bibliographical references (p.).
ISBN 0-8493-8168-1 (alk. paper)
1. Radioisotope scanning--Safety measures. I. Title.

RC78.7.R4L65 2006
616.07'575--dc22 2006047551

Visit the Taylor & Francis Web site at
http://www.taylorandfrancis.com

and the CRC Press Web site at
http://www.crcpress.com

To my students
in Oak Ridge, Tampa, and in
Central and South America —
my best wishes
wherever they may be

Preface to the Second Edition

The main objectives of this book remain unchanged in this second edition. They are to teach the students of nuclear medicine (NM) technology: (1) the principles of radiation physics, (2) the units of radioactivity, radiation exposure, and radiation dosimetry, (3) the principles of instrumentation needed for radiation detection and measurement, (4) the basis of NM imaging, (5) the scientific basis of radiation safety, (6) the rules and regulations of radiation safety, (7) the practice of radiation safety in hospitals and clinics in the United States, and (8) the fundamentals of radiobiology.

The field of NM has made many advances in the few years since this book was first published in 1999. Thanks to the efforts of the global biomedical community, those advances are making the diagnosis, the management, and the treatment of illnesses more sensitive, more specific, more accurate, and safer for patients of all ages. In this second edition, those advances are introduced keeping in mind that the final scope is the teaching of the radiological safety of the patients, the NM personnel, and all visitors to the NM department of hospitals and clinics. Some examples of those advancements follow.

1. The progress made in positron emission tomography (PET), its related radiopharmaceuticals, instrumentation, and procedures has been remarkable. This has been possible for two reasons: (1) the expansion of Medicare coverage and other insurance plans for PET imaging procedures and (2) the subsequent multiplication of medical cyclotron facilities (PET centers) in metropolitan areas. These facilities produce the necessary positron-emitting radionuclides and the labeled compounds using robotic radiochemical synthesizers.
2. The merging of two imaging modalities: (1) the metabolic images of PET using ^{18}F-labeled deoxyglucose (FDG) and (2) the exquisite anatomical images of computerized tomography (CT), in one scanning procedure lasting less than eight minutes. This combination is, without a doubt, of utmost importance to the patient.
3. Many new imaging and therapeutic radiopharmaceuticals that use "molecular targeting" as a method of localization are being tested now and soon shall become routine in NM. This should not surprise us since for years radiolabeled antibodies have been used to target specific antigens within tissues both for imaging and for treatment. The "magic bullets" and the age of molecular medicine are here to stay.

Recent revisions in the U.S. Code of Federal Regulations, Title 10, (10CFR), parts 19, 20, 30, and 35, which apply to the use of radiopharmaceuticals in medicine, are also introduced in this second edition of the book. The CFR is the document enforced by the Nuclear Regulatory Commission (NRC) in 18 states and the designated agencies in the remaining 32 "agreement states" within the U.S.

The role played by nuclear medicine technologists (NMTs) in the everyday practice of NM must be recognized. As their responsibilities become more and more complex with the arrival of new methodologies, they must participate in "on-site" training programs and in continuing education plans to earn and maintain accreditation. The efforts of the Society of Nuclear Medicine, Technology Section (SNMTS), in this regard must be recognized and appreciated, also. Its "Performance and Responsibility Guidelines for NMTs," approved at the SNM annual meeting of June 2003, is contributing to the update and upgrade of educational programs for NMTs.

The author wishes to express his gratitude to the many persons who directly or indirectly participated in making this second edition a reality. Special recognition and appreciation is given to Martin Sabarsky, vice president of corporate development, Diversa Corporation, San Diego, for his invaluable assistance in the editing of the original manuscript and in the remaking of six illustrations. My gratitude is extended also to Pete Shackett, B.A., C.N.M.T., A.R.R.T.(N), of Palmetto, Florida, and to Beverly Ammidown, C.N.M.T., of Gainesville, Florida, for their assistance in the literature research. My love goes to all the members of my family for their constant encouragement in the pursuit of this worthwhile project.

Max H. Lombardi

Author

Max H. Lombardi was born in Peru, South America. He attended primary and secondary schools in Mollendo and Lima. He earned his B.V.M. and D.V.M. degrees at the University of San Marcos in 1957 and 1958, respectively. In 1960, he earned a fellowship from the Rockefeller Foundation to study radiation biology at Cornell. The following year, he earned his M.S. degree with a major in radiation biology and minors in biochemistry and animal nutrition. He then returned to the University of San Marcos where he took the position of assistant professor.

In 1964, the Oak Ridge Institute of Nuclear Studies (ORINS) asked Dr. Lombardi to organize and coordinate the training programs of "Atoms in Action" for Latin America, an exhibit sponsored by the U.S. Atomic Energy Commission (USAEC). Between 1964 and 1969, the exhibit was successfully presented in nine countries of Central and South America. In 1965, he was asked to join the staff of ORINS as a scientist.

In 1968, Dr. Lombardi was promoted to senior scientist, assuming responsibility for the coordination of radiation biology training programs for college teachers sponsored by the National Science Foundation. At the time, he developed a number of training experiments using animals and computers and published a number of articles in the *Journal of Veterinary Research.*

In 1969, he took responsibility for the Medical Radioisotopes Qualification Course, which, under the USAEC, trained physicians in the science and practice of nuclear medicine (NM). He remained in that position until 1977. More than 1,000 physicians were trained in that period. In December of 1970, he became a U.S. citizen.

In 1977, Dr. Lombardi competed for and won the position of full-time professor of nuclear medicine at the Hillsborough Community College (HCC) in Tampa, Florida. In 1979, he earned certification by the American Board of Science in Nuclear Medicine (ABSNM). In 1982, he became director of the NMT Program and radiation safety officer of HCC, positions which he held until his retirement in 1997. During his tenure, he has trained over 300 nuclear medicine technologists.

During his career, Dr. Lombardi has participated in many conferences and continuing education programs by the Society of NM, the Florida NMT Association, the Health Physics Society, the Clinical Ligand Assays Society, the World Federation of Nuclear Medicine and Biology, and the Association of Latin American NM. He has lectured in the U.S. and twelve foreign countries. Dr. Lombardi is fluent in Spanish, English, Portuguese, and Italian. At present, he resides in San Diego, California.

Contents

Chapter 1 Principles of Radiation Physics 1

I. Rationale 1
II. Brief History of Radiation Science 1
  A. The Nature of Matter 1
  B. Atoms and Molecules 2
  C. X-Rays and Natural Radioactivity 2
  D. Relativity 3
  E. Quantum Physics 3
  F. Radiation Physics 4
III. Matter and Energy 4
  A. Nature of Matter 4
  B. Laws of Thermodynamics 4
  C. Some Basic Units 5
    1. Mass 5
    2. Distance 5
    3. Time 6
    4. Energy 6
    5. Speed of Light (c) 6
    6. Mass–Energy Equivalence ($E = mc^2$) 6
    7. Electrical Charge 6
IV. Atomic Structure and Radioactivity 6
  A. Basic Structure 6
  B. Nuclear Stability 7
  C. Radioactive Decay 8
  D. Modes of Radioactive Decay 10
    1. Alpha Decay 10
    2. Negatron Decay 11
    3. Positron Decay 13
    4. Electron Capture 14
    5. Gamma Decay 15
    6. Isomeric Transition (IT) 15
  E. Electromagnetic (EM) Radiations 16
    1. The EM Spectrum 18
V. Particle Interactions 19
  A. General Considerations 19
    1. Electrical Charge 19
    2. Momentum 19
    3. Impulse 19

B. Alpha Interactions 19
1. Trajectory 19
2. Range 20
3. Specific Ionization (S) 20
C. Beta Interactions (Positrons and Negatrons) 20
1. Trajectory 20
2. Range 20
3. Bremsstrahlung (Braking Radiation) 21
4. Backscatter 21
5. Annihilation Radiation 21
VI. Gamma Ray Interactions 21
A. General Considerations 21
B. Photoelectric Effect (τ) 21
C. Compton Effect (σ) 22
D. Pair Production (κ) 23
E. Internal Conversion (IC) 24
VII. Gamma Ray Interactions with Lead and Water 24
A. Some Properties of Lead 24
B. Some Properties of Water 24
C. Gamma Ray Attenuation 25
D. In Lead 25
E. In Water or Soft Tissue 26
Problems 26
References 26

Chapter 2 Units of Radiation Exposure and Dose 29

I. Rationale 29
II. Basic Concepts 29
A. Activity (A) 30
1. Relative Standardization 30
2. Absolute Standardization 31
B. Exposure (X) 31
C. Absorbed Dose (D) 32
D. Equivalent Dose ($H_{T,R}$) 32
E. Effective Dose (E) 33
F. Relative Biological Effectiveness (RBE) 34
III. Other Concepts 34
A. Specific Ionization 34
B. The W Value 35
C. Linear Energy Transfer (LET) 35
D. Range of Beta Particles 35
E. The f Value (rad/R) 35
IV. Specific Gamma Constant (Γ) 37
V. About S.I. Units 38

Problems 39
References 39

Chapter 3 Guidelines for Radiation Protection 41

I. Rationale 41
II. National and International Agencies 41
A. The Big Picture 41
B. National Council on Radiation Protection and Measurement 42
C. International Commission on Radiation Protection (ICRP) 42
D. International Commission on Radiation Units and Measurements 43
E. Nuclear Regulatory Commission (NRC) 43
F. Environmental Protection Agency (EPA) 43
G. Food and Drug Administration (FDA) 43
H. Department of Transportation (DOT) 44
I. Joint Commission on Accreditation of Health Organizations 45
J. Other Consulting Organizations 45
III. Radiation Safety and the Law 46
A. Objective 46
B. Philosophy 46
C. The Concept of Risk 47
D. The ALARA Policy 47
E. Method 47
F. Licensing (10CFR19.3) 48
1. General Licenses 48
2. Specific Licenses 48
IV. Types of Radiation Effects 48
A. Acute and Chronic Exposures 48
B. Deterministic Effects 48
C. Stochastic Effects 49
V. Other Concepts in Dosimetry 49
A. Committed Equivalent Dose, $H_T(\tau)$ 49
B. Committed Effective Dose, $E(\tau)$ 49
C. Annual Limit on Intake (ALI) 50
D. Derived Air Concentrations (DACs) 50
E. Deep Dose (H_d) 50
F. Shallow Dose (H_s) 50
G. Lens Dose (LD) 51
VI. Recommended Dose Limits 51
A. Occupational Dose Limits (10CFR20.1201) 51
B. General Public Dose Limits (10CFR20.1301) 51
C. Comments 51
VII. Radiation Safety Practice 52
A. Radiation Safety Officer (RSO) 52
B. Radiation Safety Committee (RSC) 52

C. Radiation Safety Program (RSP) 52
D. Quality Management Program (QMP) 52
E. The ALARA Program 52
F. Radiation Warning Signs 53
Problems 54
References 54

Chapter 4 Radiation Detection and Measurement 57

I. Rationale 57
II. Fundamentals 57
A. Principles 57
B. Detection 58
C. Radioactive Contamination 58
D. Measurement 58
E. Radiation Survey Instruments 58
1. Gas Detectors 58
2. Personal Exposure Monitors 59
3. Scintillation Detectors 59
F. Interpretation 59
III. Gas Detectors 59
A. Basic Design 59
1. Components 59
2. Ions Collected and Voltage 59
B. GM Survey Meters 61
1. Design 61
2. Scales 61
3. Wall Thickness 61
4. Gases 61
5. Error of Detection 61
6. Time Constant 62
7. Disadvantage 62
C. Calibration of GM Survey Meters 62
1. Sealed Source 62
2. Regulation 62
3. Correction Factor 62
D. Wipe-Test Counters 63
1. Design 63
2. Positive Wipes 63
E. Portable Ionization Chambers 63
1. Properties 63
2. Accuracy 63
3. Scales 63
F. Dose Calibrators 63
1. Accurate Assays 63
2. Safety 64

G. Pocket Dosimeters 64
1. Design 64
2. Operation 64
3. Applications 64
4. Advantage 64
H. Summary of Gas Detectors 65
IV. Scintillation Detectors 65
A. Basic Design 65
1. The Na(Tl) Detector 65
2. Principle 66
B. Associated Electronics 66
1. Single-Channel Analyzer (SCA) 66
2. The Window 67
3. Applications 67
4. Other Scintillation Detectors 67
V. Imaging Instrumentation 67
A. Conventional Imaging 68
1. Planar Imaging 68
2. SPECT 68
B. Pet Imaging 68
1. Metabolic Tracers 68
2. The PET Scanner 69
C. The Merging of PET and CT 69
1. Computerized Tomography (CT) 69
2. Coverage 69
3. The PET/CT Scanner 70
4. Applications 70
VI. Statistics of Counting 70
A. Types of Errors 70
1. Systematic Errors 70
2. Random Errors 70
3. Blunders 70
B. Statistical Distributions 70
1. Poisson Distribution 70
2. Gaussian Distribution 71
C. The Normal Distribution 71
1. Sample 71
2. Ranges of Confidence 71
3. The Meaning of σ_s 72
4. Practical Rules 72
5. Background Radiation 72
6. Coefficient of Variation (CV) 73
7. Standard Deviation of the Mean, $\sigma_{\bar{x}}$ 73
8. Total Counts Collected (N) 73
9. Reliability 73
10. Rejection of Data 74

VII. Making Decisions 74
A. Relative Error (τ) 74
1. Detector Performance 74
2. Is There Contamination? 75
VIII. Minimum Detectable Activity (MDA) 75
IX. Quality Assurance of Radiation Counters 76
A. Reliability 76
B. QA Tests 76
1. The Relative Error (τ) 76
2. The Reliability Factor (RF) 76
3. The Chi-Squared Test (χ^2) 77
Problems 78
References 78

Chapter 5 Radiation Safety in the Nuclear Medicine Department 81

I. Rationale 81
II. Design of the NM Department 82
A. Cold Areas 82
B. Lukewarm Areas 82
C. Warm Areas 83
D. Hot Areas 83
III. Description of Some Areas 83
A. Waiting Room and Reception 83
B. Nonimaging Procedures Room 83
1. Radioimmunoassays (RIAs) 84
2. Thyroid Uptake of Radioiodide 84
3. Schilling Test 84
4. Blood Volume Test 84
C. Control Room 84
D. Imaging Rooms 84
E. Radiopharmacy (Hot Lab) 85
IV. Molecular Medicine 86
V. The Radiation Safety Program (RSP) 89
A. General Considerations 89
B. Contents 90
VI. Radiation Safety Committee (RSC) 90
VII. Radiation Safety Officer (RSO) 90
VIII. Radioactive Materials License 91
IX. Quality Management Program (QMP) 91
A. Definition 91
B. Misadministrations 92
C. Recordable Events 92
D. Reportable Events 92

X. The ALARA Program ... 92
A. Objective ... 92
1. Inclusion ... 93
XI. The Practice of Radiation Safety ... 93
A. Authorized Users ... 93
B. Training of Personnel ... 93
C. Personnel Exposures ... 93
D. Record Keeping ... 93
E. Inspections (10CFR19.14, 10CFR30.52) ... 94
F. Reception of Radioactive Packages ... 94
G. Radiopharmaceuticals ... 95
H. Dose Calibrators ... 95
I. Laboratory Rules ... 96
J. Use of Radioactive Materials ... 96
K. Radioactive Waste Disposal ... 96
L. Laboratory Surveys ... 98
M. Sealed Sources ... 98
N. Radionuclide Therapy ... 98
O. Radiation Emergencies ... 98
Problems ... 99
References ... 100

Chapter 6 Safe Handling of Radioactivity ... 103

I. Rationale ... 103
II. Minimizing External Exposures ... 103
A. Principles ... 103
1. Quantity of Radioactivity Used ... 103
2. Time of Exposure ... 104
3. Effect of Distance ... 105
4. Effect of Shielding ... 106
III. Preventing Internal Contamination ... 110
A. Ingestion ... 110
B. Inhalation ... 110
C. Percutaneous Absorption ... 111
D. Accidental Injection ... 112
IV. Laboratory Rules ... 112
V. Radiation Hazards ... 113
A. Alpha Emitters ... 113
B. Negatron Emitters ... 114
C. Positron Emitters ... 115
D. Gamma Emitters ... 116
E. Neutrons ... 116
VI. Radionuclide Therapy ... 117
A. Radioiodine Therapy ... 117
1. Imaging of Metastases ... 117

2. Hyperthyroidism 117
3. Thyroid Ablation 117
B. Thyroid Ablation 118
C. Release of Patients 119
D. Room Decontamination 119
VII. Other Radionuclide Therapies 119
A. Phosphorus-32 119
B. Strontium-89 Chloride and ^{153}Sm-EDTMP 120
C. Yttrium-90 120
D. Iodine-125 120
E. Iodine-131 120
Problems 121
References 121

Chapter 7 Radiation Surveys and Waste Disposal 123

I. Rationale 123
II. Radiation Surveys 123
A. Preparation 123
B. Survey Practices 124
C. Selection of a Survey Instrument 124
D. Proper Operation 124
E. Surveying of Working Areas 125
F. Methods 125
III. Survey Instruments 126
A. GM Survey Meters 126
B. Alarm Monitors 126
C. Ionization Chambers 126
D. Surface Monitors 127
IV. Monitoring 128
A. Map of the Department 128
B. Method 128
C. Hot-Lab Housekeeping 129
D. Wipe-Test Monitoring 129
V. Accidental Contamination 130
A. Radioactive Spills 130
B. Decontamination 130
1. Minor Spills 130
2. Major Spills 130
3. Procedure 131
C. Release of ^{133}Xe 132
VI. Radioactive Wastes 132
A. Classes of Radioactive Wastes 132
B. Nuclear Medicine Wastes 133
1. Solid Wastes 133

2. Liquid Wastes ... 133
3. Radioactive Gases ... 133
C. Radiotoxicity ... 133
VII. Disposal of Radioactive Wastes ... 134
A. Disposal of Solid Wastes ... 134
1. Management of Wastes (10CFR20.2001) ... 134
2. Segregation by Half-Life ... 134
3. Biohazards ... 134
4. Radiopharmaceutical Remnants ... 134
5. Nuclide Generators ... 134
6. Labeling ... 135
7. Records ... 135
B. Liquid Wastes Disposal ... 135
C. Gases, Aerosols, and Volatile Radioiodine ... 135
D. Transportation of Wastes ... 136
VIII. Occupational Exposures ... 136
A. Occupational Exposure to ^{131}I ... 136
B. Occupational Exposure to ^{133}Xe ... 136
IX. The Environmental Protection Agency (EPA) ... 136
Problems ... 137
References ... 137

Chapter 8 Monitoring of Personnel Exposures ... 139

I. Rationale ... 139
II. Monitoring of Occupational Exposures ... 140
A. Dose Limits ... 140
B. Requirements ... 140
III. Reminder of Dose Limits ... 140
A. Occupational Dose Limits (10CFR20.1201) ... 140
B. Nonoccupational Dose Limits (10CFR20.1301) ... 140
IV. Monitoring Methods ... 141
A. Acceptable Methods ... 141
B. Film Badge Dosimetry ... 141
1. The Service ... 141
2. The Badge Case ... 141
3. The Film ... 142
4. The Emulsion ... 142
5. The Theory ... 143
6. Film Processing ... 143
7. Density ... 143
8. Calibration Curve ... 144
9. Advantages ... 145
10. Disadvantages ... 145
C. Thermoluminescence Dosimetry (TLD) ... 145
1. The Principle ... 145

2. The Theory ... 145
3. Quantification ... 145
4. The Service ... 146
5. Advantages of TLD ... 146
6. Disadvantages of TLD ... 146
D. Pocket Dosimeters ... 146
1. Description ... 146
2. Advantages ... 148
3. Disadvantages ... 148
E. Personal Alarm Monitors (Bleepers) ... 148
1. Description ... 148
2. Advantages ... 148
3. Disadvantages ... 148
F. OSL Dosimetry ... 148
1. Advantages ... 149
2. Disadvantages ... 149
V. Records of Personnel Dosimetry ... 149
A. Personnel Doses ... 149
B. Previous Records ... 149
C. Committed Dose ... 149
D. Other Records ... 149
VI. Reports ... 149
A. Lost or Stolen Radioactive Sources ... 149
B. Incident Reports (10CFR20.2202) ... 150
1. Immediate Notification ... 150
2. Twenty-Four-Hour Notification ... 150
VII. Reportable Events ... 150
A. Incidents ... 150
B. The EPA ... 150
C. Reports to Individuals ... 150
D. Files ... 150
Problems ... 151
References ... 151

Chapter 9 Internal Dosimetry and Bioassays ... 153

I. Rationale ... 153
II. Historical Review ... 153
A. General Considerations ... 153
B. Methods ... 154
C. The ICRP Method ... 154
1. Assumptions ... 154
2. "Standard Man" ... 154
3. The Snyder–Fisher Phantom ... 154
4. The Marinelli Equations ... 155
5. Effective Half-Life (T_e) ... 155

D. The MIRD Method 156
1. MIRD Assumptions 156
2. The MIRD Equations 157
3. Cumulative Activities ($\tilde{A}$) 157
4. Equilibrium Dose Constants (Δ_i) 157
5. Absorbed Fraction (ϕ_i) 157
6. Effective Absorbed Energies (EAE) 158
7. Mean Absorbed Doses (S) 158
8. Internal Doses According to MIRD 159
E. The Radar Web Site 159
III. Internal Doses from Radiopharmaceuticals 160
A. Package Inserts 160
1. Requirement 160
B. Diagnostic RPs 160
1. Conventional Imaging Procedures 160
2. Dosimetry of ^{18}F-FDG 160
3. Dosimetry of Radionuclide Therapy 160
4. Diagnostic Whole-Body and Fetal Doses 162
IV. Bioassay of Radioactivity 162
A. Definitions 162
B. Requirements 163
C. Airborne Medical Radionuclides 163
D. Bioassays of Iodine-131 163
1. Alert and Action Levels for ^{131}I 163
2. Action Levels 164
E. Biological Models 164
1. Highly Diffusible Radionuclides 164
2. High-Organ-Uptake Radionuclides 165
V. Biological Half-Times 166
A. Exponential Removal 166
Problems 167
References 168

Chapter 10 Introduction to Radiobiology 171

I. Rationale 171
II. Review of Basic Concepts 171
A. Living Organisms 171
B. Properties of Living Organisms 171
C. Energy Flow 172
D. Cellular Respiration 173
E. Cell Division 174
F. Mitosis 174
G. The Cell Cycle 175
H. Defense Mechanisms 175

III. The Study of Radiobiology 176
A. The General Scheme 176
B. Sources of Radiation 176
C. The Biological System 177
IV. Types of Exposure 178
A. Acute Exposure 178
B. Chronic Exposure 179
C. Experimental Levels of Exposure 179
V. Theories of Radiation Injury 179
A. Introduction 179
B. Target Theory 180
C. Indirect Theory 181
VI. DNA: The Most Sensitive Target 182
A. Lesions in DNA 182
B. Role of DNA 183
VII. Quantitative Radiobiology 184
A. Survival Curves 184
B. Microscopic Autoradiography 184
C. Other Methods 184
VIII. Survival Curves 184
A. Definition 184
B. Equations 185
C. The Shoulder 185
IX. Tissue Sensitivities 186
A. Cells 186
B. Cell Populations 186
C. The Law of Bergonie and Tribondeau 186
X. Types of Damage 186
A. Sublethal Damage (SLD) 186
B. Potentially Lethal Damage (PLD) 187
XI. Radiation Injury Modifiers 187
A. Physical Modifiers 187
B. Chemical Modifiers 187
C. Biological Modifiers 188
D. The Overkill Effect 188
E. Dose Fractionation 189
XII. Acute Radiation Syndrome (ARS) 189
A. Whole-Body Exposure 189
B. The Bone Marrow Syndrome 190
C. GI Syndrome 190
D. CNS Syndrome 191
E. Radiation Dispersion Device (RDD) 191
XIII. Late Effects of Radiation 192
A. Types of Late Effects 192
B. The Human Experience 192
C. Hypotheses for Late Effects 193

D. Radiation Hormesis 194
E. The Concept of Risk 194
F. Life-Span Shortening 196
G. Other Late Effects 196
XIV. Genetic Effects 197
A. Basic Concepts 197
B. Background Radiation 198
C. Mutations in *Drosophila* 198
D. The Megamouse Project 198
XV. Effects of Prenatal Irradiation 198
A. Experiments with Mice 198
B. Observations in Humans 199
C. Recommendations 199
Problems 199
References 200

Appendix A — Properties of Medical Radionuclides 203

A. Negatron Emitters 203
B. Gamma (X-Rays) Emitters 203
C. Positron Emitters (Annihilation Radiation) 204

Appendix B — Symbols and Abbreviations 205

Appendix C — Interconversion of Units 211

Appendix D — Answers to Problems 213

Chapter 1 213
Chapter 2 213
Chapter 3 214
Chapter 4 215
Chapter 5 215
Chapter 6 216
Chapter 7 216
Chapter 8 217
Chapter 9 217
Chapter 10 218

Index 219

1 Principles of Radiation Physics

I. RATIONALE

Radiopharmaceuticals (RPs) are radiation-emitting substances used as radiotracers in radiation biology, in biomedical research, and in the practice of nuclear medicine (NM). There is no question about the usefulness of radiotracers in these fields of science. In the hands of well-trained persons, radiotracers are wonderful tools that can save time and effort in solving problems. When improperly used, however, radioactive materials can result in unnecessary exposures to personnel, patients, and visitors to the NM department of a hospital or clinic.

To comprehend the hazards of radiation and to avoid unnecessary exposures, we must first understand the nature and properties of those radiations: how they are emitted and how they interact with materials such as lead, the most important shielding material, and with the human body. This chapter begins with a review of the history of radiation science. In this manner we honor the pioneers who laid the foundations of modern science, including NM. That is followed by a review of the nature and properties of those radiations that are of immediate concern in the practice of NM.

II. BRIEF HISTORY OF RADIATION SCIENCE

A. The Nature of Matter

From 530 to 240 B.C.E., Greek philosophers developed their own ideas about the nature of matter. Pythagoras explained that matter was made of four elements: earth, water, air, and fire. Their properties were hot, cold, wet, and dry. Democritus proposed that matter was discontinuous, made of tiny, indivisible particles, which he called *atoms*, and the rest, he said, was vacuum. Aristotle later endorsed Pythagoras's hypothesis. However, Pythagoras is best known for his theorem of rectangular triangles: $c^2 = a^2 + b^2$. In 240 B.C.E., Archimedes was the first to measure the density of solids. He discovered the principle of buoyancy, according to which a body submerged in a fluid is lifted by a buoyant force equal to the weight of the fluid displaced. Supposedly, he discovered it while taking a bath. He then ran, yelling, "eureka, eureka" — "I found it! I found it!"

B. Atoms and Molecules

For over 2000 years, the ideas of the Greek philosophers were accepted as facts. But in 1780, Antoine Lavoisier announced the law of conservation of mass, which holds that in any physical or chemical reaction, the mass of the products must be equal to the mass of the reactants. No mysterious appearances or disappearances were possible. Lavoisier also studied the composition of air and discovered the role of oxygen in respiration and in the combustion of matter. For these and other discoveries, Lavoisier is considered to be the father of chemistry.

In 1808, John Dalton proposed the law of multiple proportions, which provides that when two or more elements combine to form other compounds, one of them remains constant and the others vary in proportion to the simple digits 1, 2, 3, etc. For example, hydrogen and oxygen make H_2O and H_2O_2, water and hydrogen peroxide, respectively. For this reason, Dalton is considered to be the first to offer proof of the existence of atoms. In 1811, Amadeus Avogadro defined atoms and molecules. He discovered "Avogadro's number" — 6.023×10^{23}, which is the number of atoms in a gram atom weight of any element or the number of molecules in a gram molecular weight of any compound. Avogadro's number is a universal constant.

Henrich Geissler in 1854 investigated electrical discharges in vacuum tubes. Forty years later, J.J. Thomson discovered that those "cathode rays" in Geissler's tubes were made of tiny negatively charged particles, which he called *electrons*. In 1898, Thomson proposed his first model of the atom: "Atoms are made of spheres of positive electrical charge balanced by equally spaced negative charges (electrons) within." In 1911, Ernest Rutherford, experimenting on the scattering of alpha particles by gold foil, discovered the atomic nucleus. He proposed the nuclear model of the atom: "Most of the atom is empty space; the positive charge is concentrated in a very small nucleus; electrons move around in orbits."

In 1932, James Chadwick discovered the neutron. His discovery explained the mystery of isotopes-atoms of the same element having different atomic weights. The same year, Anderson discovered the *positron* — a positively charged electron emitted by some radioactive nuclides. Positrons are the "antimatter" of negative electrons. The same year, Cocroft and Walton invented the linear accelerator, and Lawrence invented the cyclotron, both useful tools in the study of atomic and nuclear structure. Two years later, in 1934, Frederick Joliot and Irene Curie (daughter of Madam Curie) discovered artificial radioactivity.

C. X-Rays and Natural Radioactivity

In 1895, Wilhelm Roentgen, working with vacuum tubes and fluorescent screens, serendipitously discovered x-rays. The following year, Becquerel discovered in a similar fashion natural radioactivity in some uranium rocks. In 1898, Marie and Pierre Curie discovered polonium and radium, two radioactive elements. The emissions of these elements were named alpha, beta, and gamma radiations.

D. Relativity

In 1905, Albert Einstein proposed two postulates: (a) the principle of relativity, which basically said that the laws of physics are the same for all observers in uniform motion, and (b) the constancy of the speed of light: the speed of light is the same to observers moving relative to each other. This theory abolished the Newtonian concept of absolute space and time. It also disposed of the Maxwellian concept of the "ether," which was supposed to be the medium needed for the propagation of light. In a separate publication, Einstein famously added the principle of equivalence between mass and energy: $E = mc^2$.

In 1916, Einstein proposed his general theory of relativity, a theory of gravity. Basically, the theory states that (a) gravity and acceleration are one and the same, (b) the laws of physics are the same in all frames of reference, not only those in uniform motion, (c) space–time is curved, and gravity is a manifestation of curved space–time (the geometry of space–time), (d) the curvature of space–time is more pronounced near a large mass, such as a star or a galaxy, and (e) light is bent as it follows the curves of space–time. Recent discoveries show that galaxies behave as gravitational lenses that produce multiple images of objects behind them. The theory also predicts the existence of objects so dense that they curve space–time so much that not even light can escape them (black holes). Time dilatation, mass increase, and space contraction in the direction of motion, observed at relativistic velocities, are some of the consequences of the theory of general relativity.

E. Quantum Physics

In 1900, Max Planck introduced what became known as quantum theory: Electromagnetic radiations are emitted and absorbed in discrete amounts of energy which he called *quanta* (plural of quantum). In 1905, Albert Einstein explained the photoelectric effect (PE), by which light impinging upon a metal plate removes electrons from it. He added that the photoelectric effect proves that electromagnetic (EM) radiations are emitted and absorbed in quanta. He named a quantum of EM radiation a *photon*, an entity having dual nature: properties of particles and properties of waves. In 1913, Niels Bohr proposed the quantum model of the atom: electrons move in circular orbits corresponding to well-defined (discrete) levels of energy. The number of orbits is restricted by a quantized angular momentum. While in orbit, electrons do not emit radiation, and their energy level is characterized by the principal quantum number "n," which assumes values of 1, 2, 3, etc. Emission or absorption of energy occurs only when an electron jumps from one orbit to another (quantum jumps). In 1916, Arnold Sommerfeld proposed that electrons move in elliptical orbits and that, to describe their motion, two quantum numbers were needed: n, the principal quantum number and "k," the angular momentum quantum number (later renamed "l"). In 1925, Uhlembeck, Goutsmit, and others proposed "m," the magnetic quantum number to describe the angular momentum of electrons in an externally applied magnetic field, and "s," the spin quantum number, to explain the splitting of spectral lines in magnetic fields. Then came De Broglie, who proposed that particles behave as waves too and that electrons have shorter wavelengths than light.

The same year, Wolfgang Pauli proposed his exclusion principle: in an atom, no two electrons can have the same combination of quantum numbers. The following year, Schroedinger proposed that electron orbits are more like probability curves of space–time. He named them *orbitals*. In 1927, Heissenberg proposed his principle of uncertainty: the position and the momentum of a particle cannot be determined simultaneously. If one of them is determined, the other can only be expressed in terms of probabilities. This concept abolished the strict determinism of the Newtonian (predictable) "clock universe."

F. Radiation Physics

In 1919, Ernest Rutherford converted nitrogen into oxygen by bombardment with alpha radiation. This was the first time that an element had been artificially converted into another (transmutation). In 1923, Arthur Compton explained mathematically the coherent scattering of photons, now known as the Compton Effect. The scattered photons have well-defined energies that depend on the angle of deflection. In 1934, Enrico Fermi described the transmutation of elements by neutron capture. He also named the small particle that accompanies beta decay as "neutrino."

Hahn and Strassman discovered nuclear fission in 1939. The same year, Fermi proposed the possibility of a controlled fission chain reaction. In 1942, Fermi and his team achieved just that in a "pile" of graphite and enriched uranium fuel elements built under the stands of the football stadium of the University of Chicago. This was the first manmade nuclear reactor. The following year, Fermi and his team built a second graphite reactor at the Oak Ridge National Laboratory in Tennessee. That reactor supplied the world with radioisotopes for industry and medicine for many years.

III. MATTER AND ENERGY

A. Nature of Matter

Matter is made of atoms; atoms are made of subatomic particles bound together by nuclear and electromagnetic forces. Atoms bind to other atoms to make molecules. Molecules join other molecules to make crystals, fibers, cells, tissues, organs, and organisms. The association and dissociation of atoms and molecules involve energy transfers: absorption and emission of energy. Besides the nuclear, strong, weak, and EM forces, the gravitational force completes the set of forces of nature, which make the universe the way it is. A recent theory has joined the EM force with the nuclear weak force: the electroweak force. Table 1.1 summarizes the forces of nature. Matter is "frozen energy," as demonstrated by Einstein with his equation $E = mc^2$. As we will see, positron emission and positron annihilation are remarkable proofs of that statement. In the NM department, we experience that proof every time a PET (positron emission tomography) scan is done on a patient.

B. Laws of Thermodynamics

All transfers of energy in physical, chemical, and biological systems comply with the laws of thermodynamics. A brief description follows.

TABLE 1.1
The Forces of Nature

Force	Binds	Examples
Strong nuclear	Protons and neutrons	Nuclear fission and fusion
Weak nuclear	Quarks within nucleons	Neutron–proton interconversions in beta decay
EM force	Atoms together to make molecules, crystals	Electrical and magnetic phenomena, chemical bonding
Gravity	All matter in the universe	Motion of planets, stars, and galaxies

1. *First law*: This is the law of conservation of mass or energy, which says that, in all phenomena, energy can be converted from one form to another, but it cannot be either created or destroyed. That law was first described by Lavoisier (see the preceding section on history).
2. *Second law*: This is the law of energy flow, which says that all spontaneous processes are capable of doing work. That means that, in spontaneous processes, energy flows from high-energy states to low-energy states. When this happens, energy is released. That energy can be put to work. For example, burning coal is the oxidation of carbon to form carbon dioxide; in the process, heat and light are released. In spontaneous processes, entropy increases. Entropy is a measure of the degree of disorder. When energy is released, entropy (disorder) increases.
3. *Third law*: This is the law of entropy, which says that, at absolute zero, the entropy of a pure crystal is zero. Although pure crystals and absolute zero are very difficult to achieve, they are considered properties of perfection in nature and manifestations of the highest energy state.

C. Some Basic Units

1. Mass

The gram (g) is defined as one-thousandth of the S.I. (international system) unit, the kilogram (kg). The Dalton (Da) or atomic mass unit (amu) = 1.66×10^{-27} kg.

2. Distance

The meter (m) is defined as the distance equal to 1,650,767.73 wavelengths of the orange light emitted by ^{86}Kr in a vacuum. The subunits of the meter are

Centimeter (cm) = 10^{-2} m
Millimeter = 10^{-3} m
Micron (μm) = 10^{-6} m
Angstrom (Å) = 10^{-10} m

3. Time

The second (s) is the S.I. unit of time and is equal to the duration of 9,192,631,770 periods (wavelengths) of the radiation emitted between two hyperfine lines in the Cs spectrum.

4. Energy

In the macroworld, the MKS system (meter, kilogram, second) is used. The unit of energy is the joule (J), which is equal to the force of a newton (N) acting over a distance of 1 m. One N is the force that gives a mass of 1 kg an acceleration of 1 m/s each second: $J = kg - m/s^2$.

In the microworld, the unit of energy is the electron volt (eV), which is equal to the kinetic energy gained by an electron when accelerated across a potential difference of 1 V. Multiples are keV = 10^3 eV, MeV = 10^6 eV, and GeV = 10^9 eV.

5. Speed of Light (c)

$c = 3 \times 10^8$ m/s in a vacuum, the same for all EM radiations (a universal constant).

6. Mass–Energy Equivalence ($E = mc^2$)

$$\text{electron mass } (m_e) = 9.11 \times 10^{-31} \text{ kg; and } c^2 = (3 \times 10^8 \text{ m/s})^2$$

$$mc^2 = (9.11 \times 10^{-31} \text{ kg})(3 \times 10^8 \text{ m/s})^2 = 8.2 \times 10^{-14} \text{ J}$$

$$8.2 \times 10^{-14} \text{ J}/1.6 \times 10^{-13} \text{ J/MeV} = 0.511 \text{ MeV}$$

$$1 \text{ atomic mass unit (Da)} = 1.66 \times 10^{-27} \text{ kg} = 931 \text{ MeV}$$

7. Electrical Charge

One unit of electrostatic electrical charge = 1.6×10^{-19} C and is the same for all electrons. Protons carry the same charge, but are positive.

IV. ATOMIC STRUCTURE AND RADIOACTIVITY

A. Basic Structure

1. Atoms are very small. Their diameters vary between 1 and 5 Å.
2. Electrons move in orbitals around the nucleus of the atom. They carry one unit of electrical charge, which is negative.
3. The nucleus is extremely small. Its diameter is about 10^{-4} Å, or 10^{-14} m.
4. The nucleus contains protons (p) and neutrons (n). Protons carry one unit of electrical charge, positive. Neutrons carry no charge. Table 1.2 gives the properties of the three basic atomic particles.

TABLE 1.2
Basic Atomic Particles

Particle	Mass in Da	Electrical Charge
Proton (p)	1.0079	+1
Neutron (n)	1.0090	0
Electron (e)	0.0005	–1

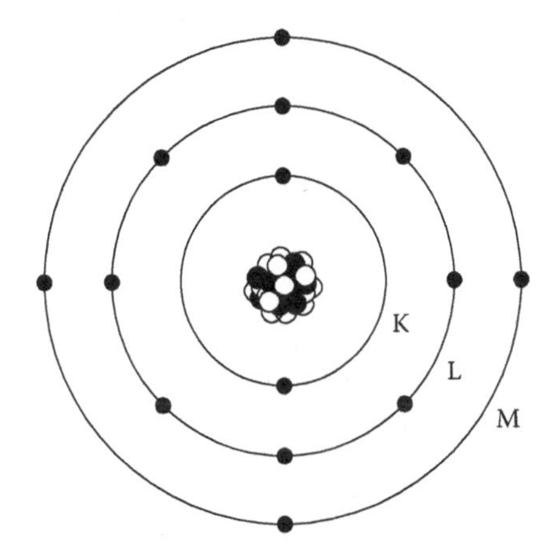

FIGURE 1.1 Model of the atom. The nucleus contains protons and neutrons. Electron orbitals K, L, and M are shown. Nuclear forces bind the nucleons in the nucleus. EM forces bind the electron orbitals to the nucleus.

5. In recent years, scientists have proposed the theory of "the standard model" of the atom, which considers that protons and neutrons are made of "up" and "down" quarks. In this book, we need not discuss that theory. Some of the references at the end of this chapter describe those concepts.
6. Figure 1.1 shows a very schematic model of the atom, the "planetary system model." This model is certainly imperfect, because it shows only two dimensions. However, models such as this help us understand the properties of matter.

B. Nuclear Stability

1. An attractive strong nuclear force is postulated to exist between neutrons, between neutrons and protons, and even between protons and protons.
2. That force is many times stronger than the repulsive electrical force between the protons. It is the binding force of the nucleus.
3. The nuclear force is "short range." It can be felt only at a distance of one nuclear radius.
4. An element is characterized by the number of protons in the nucleus, which equals its atomic number Z.

5. Atoms of the same element having different number of neutrons are called isotopes of that element. They have different masses; for example, ^{123}I, ^{125}I, ^{127}I, and ^{131}I are isotopes of the element iodine — all have 53 protons in the nucleus, but they differ in the number of neutrons. Because they all have the same electronic configuration, they have the same chemical properties.
6. The stability of a nucleus appears to be related to the n/p ratio in the nucleus. Some of those isotopes mentioned above may have an n/p ratio different from the one needed for stability. They are radioactive or radioisotopes of that element.
7. A nuclide is any combination of neutrons and/or protons that lives long enough to be detected. A radionuclide is a radioactive nuclide. By definition, a free proton is a nuclide. Also, a free neutron is a nuclide. Actually, neutrons are radionuclides because they decay to protons by emitting beta particles. Their half-life is about 12 min.

C. Radioactive Decay

1. Radioactivity is the spontaneous transformation of atomic nuclei accompanied by the emission of energy in the form of particles and/or photons.
2. The special unit of radioactivity, or activity for short, is the curie (Ci), which is equal to 3.7×10^{10} nuclear transformations per second (nt/s). See Chapter 2 for details on units.
3. The period in which the activity of a source decays to one-half of its original value is the half-life ($t_{1/2}$).
4. The activity (A) of a source is proportional to the number of radioactive atoms (N), and the proportionality constant is the decay constant (α):

$$A = \lambda N \tag{1.1}$$

where A = activity in nt/s; λ = fraction of N decaying/s; and N = number of radioactive atoms.

5. The decay constant expresses the rate of decay or the fraction of atoms decaying per unit time. The decay constant is characteristic of each radionuclide and remains truly constant in all physical, chemical, and biological phenomena. This is one of the reasons radiotracers are so useful in biomedical research and in NM.
6. The decay constant and the half-life are related by the following equation:

$$\lambda = 0.693/t_{1/2} \tag{1.2}$$

where 0.693 = ln 2 (the natural log of 2).

7. The activity of a source decreases exponentially with time. The remaining activity after some time t can be calculated with the following equation:

$$A_t = A_o e^{-\lambda t} \quad (1.3)$$

where A_t = activity at some time t; A_o = original activity; e = base of natural logs; λ = decay constant; and t = elapsed time.

8. The mean life (τ) of the radioactive atoms in a source is the sum of all the lives divided by the number of atoms. Statistically, it can be shown that

$$\tau = 1/\lambda = 1.443t_{1/2} \quad (1.4)$$

9. Table 1.3 gives the half-lives of most commonly used medical radionuclides grouped by mode of decay. Figure 1.2 shows the decay of a sample of ^{99m}Tc (half-life of 6 h).

TABLE 1.3
Half-Lives of Medical Radionuclides

Mode of Decay	Radionuclide	Half-Life
Negatron emitters	^{32}P	14.3 d
	$^{90}Sr/^{90}Y$	28 y/64 h
	^{89}Sr	50.5 d
	^{186}Re	3.8 d
	^{188}Re	16.8 h
Negatron-gamma emitters	^{131}I	8.05 d
	^{133}Xe	5.3 d
	^{99}Mo	66 h
	^{137}Cs	30 y
Positron emitters	^{18}F	110 min
	^{11}C	20.4 min
	^{13}N	10 min
	^{15}O	2 min
	^{68}Ga	68 min
	^{82}Rb	75 sec
Isomeric transition	^{99m}Tc	6 h
	^{117m}Sn	13.6 d
Electron capture-gamma	^{123}I	13.1 h
	^{125}I	60 d
	^{111}In	2.8 d
	^{201}Tl	73 h
	^{57}Co	270 d
	^{67}Ga	78 h
	^{51}Cr	28 d

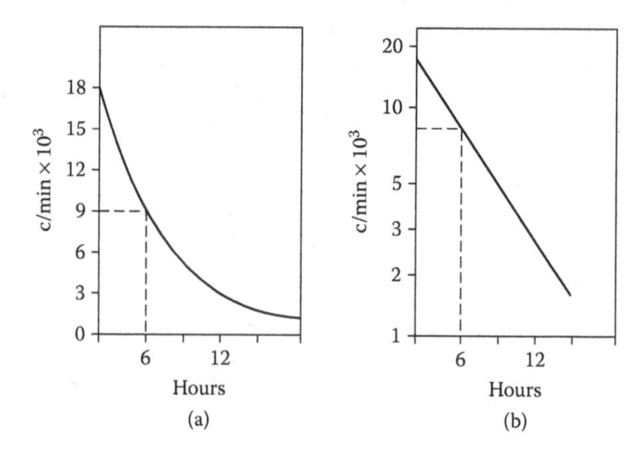

FIGURE 1.2 (a) Exponential decay of a ^{99m}Tc source. (b) When plotted on semilogarithmic graph paper, the curve becomes a straight line. The slope of the curve is the decay constant.

Sample Problems

(a) What is the number of atoms in 1 MBq (megabecquerel = 10^6 nt/s) of ^{99m}Tc?
Solution: From Equation 1.1, $N = A/\lambda$ and $\lambda = 0.693/t_{1/2}$.
Therefore, $N = (1 \times 10^6$ nt/s$)/(0.693/21{,}600$ s$)$, where 1×10^6 nt/s = definition of MBq and 21,600 is the half-life of ^{99m}Tc in seconds. $N = 5 \times 10^{10}$ atoms (answer).

(b) What is the rate of decay of ^{125}I?
Solution: That is the same as asking for the decay constant; therefore, $\lambda = 0.693/60$ d $= 0.01155$/d or 1.15%/d (answer).

(c) What is the mean life of ^{99m}Tc atoms?
Solution: Equation 1.4 says that $\tau = 1.443t_{1/2}$; therefore, mean life = 1.443 × 6 h = 8.658 h (answer).

(d) A ^{99m}Tc generator arrives on Monday at 8:00 a.m. containing 22 GBq of ^{99}Mo. What is its activity at 8:00 a.m. on Tuesday?
Solution: Equation 1.3 allows us to state that the activity at 24 h will be $A_t = 22\ e^{-(0.693 \times 24/66)}$. $A_t = 17.1$ GBq (answer).

D. Modes of Radioactive Decay

The classic approach of describing nuclear radiations as alpha, beta (positrons and negatrons), and gamma radiations is followed here. X-ray emissions are consequential to electron capture (EC) and internal conversion (IC) modes of decay.

1. Alpha Decay

Alpha particle emission is a stabilizing process of nuclei having too many nucleons (neutrons and protons). Alpha particles have a mass of 4 Da and a charge of +2 units; therefore, they are equivalent to helium-4 ions (He^{2+}). Alpha particles, emitted

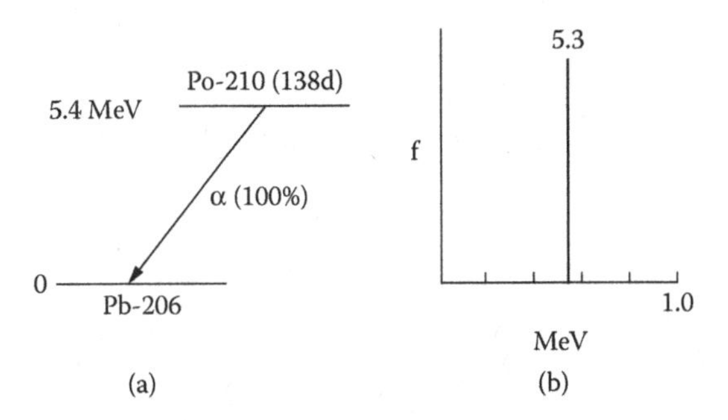

FIGURE 1.3 (a) Polonium-210 decays by alpha emission to lead-206. (b) The alpha spectrum shows that alpha particles are monoenergetic. See also Figure 6.7.

by radionuclides, have energies in the range of 1.8 to 11.7 MeV. Upon emission, alpha particles travel with a speed of about 1/30c.

Artificial "alphas" (He ions) can be accelerated to energies reaching many GeV (giga-electron-volt, or 10^9 eV). For a given transition, alphas are monoenergetic. The spectrum (a graph of frequency or number vs. energy) shows a discrete line. Figure 1.3(a) shows the decay scheme of polonium-210, which emits 5.3 MeV alpha particles; Figure 1.3(b) shows their spectrum. Upon emission, the daughter ^{206}Pb carries 0.1 MeV of recoil energy:

$$^{210}\text{Po} \rightarrow {}^{206}\text{Pb} + {}^{4}\text{He} + 5.4\text{ MeV}$$

$$(0.1\text{ MeV})\ (5.3\text{ MeV})$$

Decay schemes are graphs of energy level vs. atomic number. Alpha emitters are not used in medicine. Most of them are heavy metals unsuitable for diagnostic applications. However, some exceptional therapeutic applications are found in the medical literature.

2. Negatron Decay

Negatron emission is a stabilizing process of nuclei having more neutrons than those needed for stability. Negatrons (represented by the symbol β^-) have the same mass and electrical charge of orbital electrons, but they originate in the nucleus at the very instant of decay. In negatron decay, a neutron is converted into a proton. The daughter has one more proton than the parent (Z increases by one unit). The mass does not change significantly. Every negatron emitted is accompanied by an antineutrino represented by the symbol $\bar{\nu}$.

Negatrons have energies in the range of a few kiloelectronvolts to 14 MeV. Upon emission, they travel with a speed of about 1/3 c. For a given transition, negatrons have a continuum spectrum of energies. The average energy ($\bar{E}_\beta$) is about 1/3 of the maximum energy (E_{max}) available.

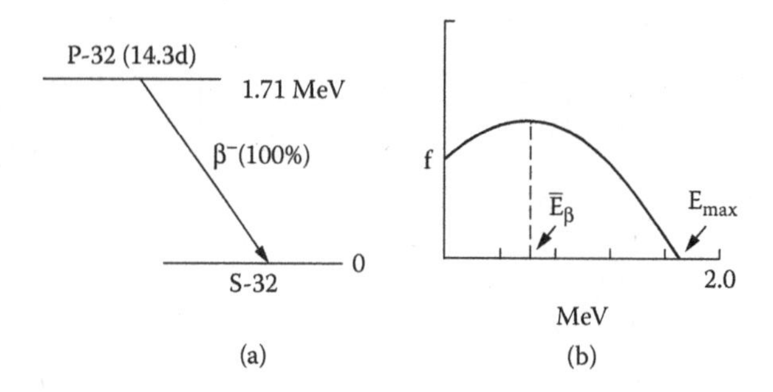

FIGURE 1.4 (a) Phosphorus-32 decays by negatron emission to sulfur-32. (b) The spectrum shows that the negatrons have a continuum of energies up to a maximum (E_{max}) of 1.71 MeV. The average energy is about 1/3 of E_{max}.

Figure 1.4(a) shows the decay scheme of ^{32}P, and Figure 1.4(b) shows its negatron spectrum. The continuum spectrum is explained by the simultaneous emission of an antineutrino that shares the E_{max} with the negatron. The antineutrino has a very small mass, with only 0.0005 of the mass of an electron. For that reason, antineutrinos fly at almost the speed of light. For the example of Figure 1.4, the reaction is

$$^{32}P \rightarrow {}^{32}S + {}_{-1}\beta + \bar{\nu}$$

Most negatron emitters are reactor-produced. They are important in NM, particularly in radionuclide therapy. For example, ^{32}P, ^{89}Sr, and ^{153}Sm, among others, are used in palliation of pain in cases of metastatic bone cancer. ^{32}P, as a phosphate, is also used in the treatment of polycythemia and, as a colloidal suspension, in the therapy of intracavitary malignant disease. Another example is ^{90}Y, which, when bound to a monoclonal antibody, is used to treat non-Hodgkins lymphoma (NHL). ^{131}I, a negatron-gamma emitter, is used in the therapy of hyperthyroidism and cancer of the thyroid gland. Table 1.4 shows the basic physical properties of negatron emitters in NM. See also Table 6.3.

TABLE 1.4
Negatron Emitters in Nuclear Medicine

Radionuclide	$t_{1/2}$	E_{max} (keV)	Range in Water (mm)
^{32}P	14.3 d	1710	8.0
^{89}Sr	50.5 d	1491	6.6
^{186}Re	3.8 d	1077	4.3
^{188}Re	16.8 h	1965	10.0
^{153}Sm	1.9 d	702	2.5
^{177}Lu	6.7 d	497	1.5
^{90}Sr	28 y	546	1.75
^{90}Y	64 h	2384	12.2

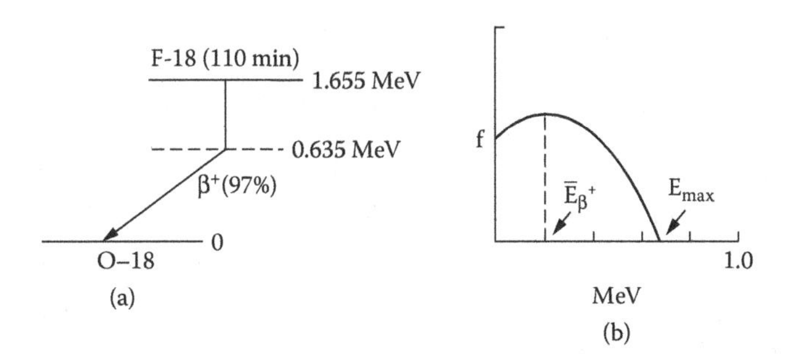

FIGURE 1.5 (a) Fluorine-18 decays by positron emission to oxygen-18. The vertical line on the decay scheme represents the 1.02 MeV of energy needed for positron decay. (b) The spectrum shows that positrons have a continuum of energies up to a maximum (E_{max}) of 635 keV. The average energy is about 1/3 of E_{max}.

3. Positron Decay

Positron emission is a stabilizing process of nuclei having fewer neutrons than those needed for stability. We could also say that it is a stabilizing process of nuclei having excess protons. But most important is that the available energy for the transition must exceed 1.02 MeV. That energy is needed for the creation of two electrons, one positive and one negative, in the nucleus, at the moment of decay. The positive electron (positron, represented by the symbols β^+ and e^+) is emitted. The negative electron joins a proton to make a neutron. Any excess energy above 1.02 MeV is shared by the positron and a neutrino (ν). That energy represents the E_{max}. Positrons are antielectrons. They have the same mass as electrons and the same electrical charge, but are positive. Their energies vary between 0.1 and 14 MeV. Upon emission, they travel with a speed of about 1/3 c. For a given transition, positrons have a continuum spectrum of energies up to a maximum, the E_{max}. The average energy is about 1/3 of E_{max}. Figure 1.5(a) shows the decay scheme of ^{18}F. The vertical line represents the 1.02 MeV of energy spent in the creation of the two electrons at the very instant of decay, and the oblique line represents the emission of the positron. Figure 1.5(b) shows the spectrum of ^{18}F positrons. The reaction is

$$^{18}F \rightarrow {}^{18}O + \beta^+ + \nu$$

In positron decay, the atomic number Z decreases by one unit. Because of their negligible mass, neutrinos travel with the speed of light. When a positron spends all its energy as it travels through matter, it comes to a stop. At this point, it attracts a free electron and, because they are antiparticles with regard to each other, they undergo annihilation. That means that their masses are converted into two 511-keV photons of EM energy emitted in exactly opposite directions. Those photons are known as *annihilation radiation*, and they are the very ones detected in PET. This phenomenon is a classic example of $E = mc^2$, in which matter is converted into energy.

Most positron emitters are produced in accelerators. In NM, they are produced in medical cyclotrons, where a target compound is irradiated with fast particles such as protons, deuterons, tritons, or helium ions. In the process, one or two nuclear

TABLE 1.5
Positron Emitters in Nuclear Medicine

Radionuclide	$t_{1/2}$	E_{max} (keV)	Range in Water (mm)
^{18}F	110 min	634	2.4
^{11}C	20.4 min	960	5.0
^{13}N	10 min	1199	5.4
^{15}O	2 min	1732	8.2
^{68}Ga	68 min	1899	9.1
^{82}Rb	75 sec	3356	15.6

particles are ejected. The product, or daughter, is the positron emitter of interest. For example, the following nuclear reaction is used in the production of ^{18}F:

$$^{16}O\ (^{3}He,\ ^{1}H)\ ^{18}F$$

In this reaction, ^{16}O is the target nucleus, ^{3}He ions are the cyclotron "bullets," ^{1}H is a proton (the ejected particle), and ^{18}F is the product of interest in NM. Table 1.5 shows the properties of positron emitters of interest in NM.

4. Electron Capture

Electron capture (EC) is a stabilizing process of nuclei having too many protons. This mode of decay competes with positron emission. The difference lies in the fact that, if the energy available for the transition is greater than 1.02 MeV, then the radionuclide may decay by either positron emission or by EC. If, on the other hand, the energy available is less than 1.02 MeV, then the only possible mode of decay is EC. There is some evidence that the K-electron oscillates through the nucleus to form the s orbital. That may explain why the K-electron has the highest probability of being captured. L-capture and M-capture occur with lower probabilities. EC results in the conversion of a proton into a neutron in the nucleus; thus, the atomic number Z decreases by one unit. EC is accompanied by the emission of a neutrino as shown in the following example of EC:

$$^{123}I + e^{-} \rightarrow {}^{123}Te + \nu$$

Many EC radionuclides emit immediately a gamma ray (prompt gamma). All EC radionuclides emit characteristic x-rays and/or Auger electrons. In NM, at least two radionuclides emit x-rays, which are more abundant than the gamma rays and have suitable energies for measurement. Those radionuclides are as follows:

a. Iodine-125, which emits 35-keV gamma rays (7%) and 27–32 keV tellurium K-x-rays (136%). 93% of the gamma rays are lost to internal conversion. ^{125}I is used in laboratory radioimmunoassays (RIAs) and in radionuclide therapy.

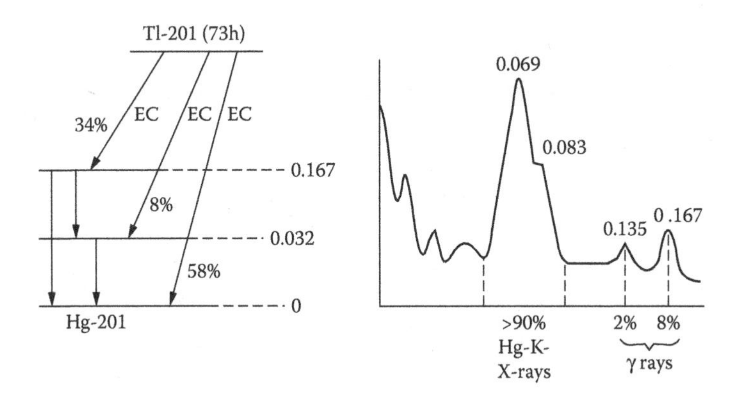

FIGURE 1.6 Thallium-201 decays by electron capture to mercury-201 (left). The main peak of the spectrum (right) represents the daughter K-x-rays with energies of 69–83 keV. Two gamma rays with energies of 135 and 167 keV are also shown.

b. Thallium-201, decays by EC and emits 135 keV (2%) and 167 keV (8%) gamma rays plus 69-83 keV Mercury K-x-rays (94%). ^{201}Tl is used as a potassium analog and, until recently, was used extensively in myocardial perfusion imaging. Figure 1.6 shows the decay scheme of ^{201}Tl and its gamma spectrum.

Most EC radionuclides are produced by cyclotrons. They are considered pure gamma emitters, which makes them ideal for diagnostic applications in NM. For example, ^{111}In bound to chelating agents and to antibodies has multiple applications, as shown in Table 5.3.

5. Gamma Decay

Gamma rays are high-energy, high-frequency EM radiations emitted by atomic nuclei following other modes of decay when the daughter nucleus still has some excitation energy available. Figure 1.7(a) gives the decay scheme of ^{111}In as an example of a gamma emitter after EC decay. Figure 1.7(b) shows its gamma spectrum. Two gamma peaks are noticeable: 173 keV (89%) and 247 keV (94%). Table 1.6 gives some gamma emitters of interest in NM, their modes of decay, and their gamma emissions with percentage abundances. Some important x-ray emissions are also shown. Gamma emitters are very important in diagnostic NM because, in the proper chemical form, they result in functional images of tissues and organ systems. Positron emitters are also considered gamma emitters because of the two annihilation gamma rays produced upon decay. Positron emission tomography (PET) produces metabolic images of the heart, the brain, and tumors in many NM imaging procedures. Table 4.4 gives the indications of some PET applications.

6. Isomeric Transition (IT)

When an excited nucleus de-excites by emission of a delayed gamma ray, the daughter is a nuclear isomer of the parent, and the process is called IT decay. Nuclear isomers

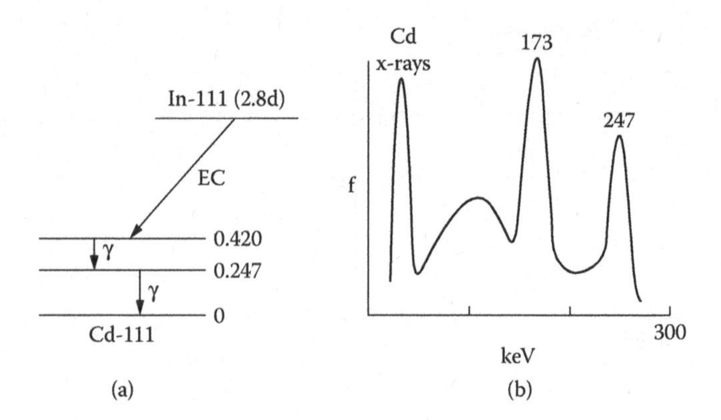

FIGURE 1.7 (a) Indium-111 decays by electron capture to cadmium-111. (b) The spectrum shows the two gamma rays emitted with energies of 173 and 247 keV and a lower energy peak from the K-x-rays of cadmium.

TABLE 1.6
Gamma Emitters in Nuclear Medicine

Nuclide	Mode of Decay	X-Rays, keV (%)	Gamma Rays, keV (%)
^{125}I	EC, gamma	Te-K-x, 27-32 (136)	35 (7)
^{133}Xe	Negatron, gamma	Cs-K-x, 32 (48)	81 (36)
^{201}Tl	EC, gamma	Hg-K-x, 69-83 (94)	135 (2), 167 (8)
^{57}Co	EC, gamma	—	123 (89), 136 (11)
^{99m}Tc	IT, gamma	—	140 (89)
^{123}I	EC, gamma	—	159 (84)
^{111}In	EC, gamma	—	173 (89), 247 (94)
^{67}Ga	EC, gamma	—	93 (40), 184 (24), 296 (22)
^{51}Cr	EC, gamma	—	320 (9)
^{99}Mo	Negatron, gamma	—	740 (12), 780 (4)
^{131}I	Negatron, gamma	—	364 (83), 638 (9)
^{137}Cs	Negatron, gamma	—	662 (84)

have the same number of protons and the same number of neutrons; only the daughter has them arranged in a more stable configuration. Figure 1.8 shows the decay scheme of ^{99m}Tc decaying to ^{99}Tc, its isomer, with a half-life of 6 h. The "m" in the symbol of ^{99m}Tc stands for metastable which means "changing into a more stable configuration." Figure 1.8 also shows the gamma spectrum of ^{99m}Tc. Technetium-99m is a most important radionuclide because it behaves as a pure gamma emitter of most suitable energy (140 keV). Table 5.2 shows a number ^{99m}Tc applications.

E. Electromagnetic (EM) Radiations

Gamma rays and x-rays are EM radiations. EM radiations represent energy emitted or absorbed in the form of photons. Photons are the carriers of discrete amounts, or

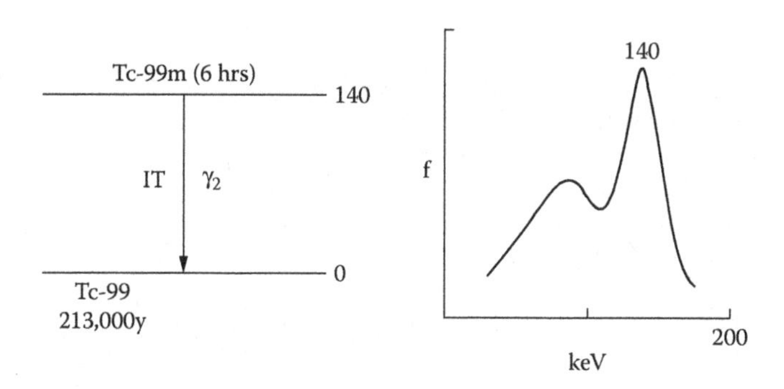

FIGURE 1.8 Technetium-99m decays by isomeric transition to technetium-99 (left). The main peak of the spectrum (right), with an energy of 140 keV, represents the delayed gamma ray emitted.

quanta, of EM energy. Photons have a dual nature; that is, they have the properties of both particles and waves. Properties of particles are their interactions by elastic and inelastic collisions. Properties of waves are reflection, refraction, dispersion, diffraction, and polarization. The general properties of photons are the following:

1. Propagation: They propagate through space in the form of waves represented by the oscillation of two fields, one electrical and one magnetic, having equal wavelengths and perpendicular to each other.
2. Speed: They propagate with the speed of light (c) in a vacuum, $c = 3 \times 10^8$ m/s.
3. Vacuum: They propagate in vacuum.
4. Momentum: They carry energy and momentum.
5. Wavelength: The speed of light, c, is a universal constant. It is essential in calculations of wavelengths and frequencies of EM radiations. The basic equations are

$$c = \lambda \nu$$

$$E = h\nu$$

$$\text{keV} = 12.4/\text{Å}$$

where c = speed of light in vacuum in m/s; λ = wavelength in m/cycle; E = energy in keV, MeV, or joules; h = Planck's Constant = 4.14×10^{-21} MeV-s, = 4.14×10^{-18} keV-s, = 6.63×10^{-34} J-s; ν = frequency in cycles/s (hertz or Hz); and Å = wavelength in angstroms (1 Å = 10^{-10} m).

Note: Universal constants mentioned in this book are Avogadro's number (N), the speed of light in vacuum (c), Planck's constant (h), the base of the natural logarithms (e), and the ratio of the length of a circle's circumference to its diameter (π).

Sample Problems

(a) What is the energy of a 1-Å x-ray?
Solution: keV = 12.4/1 Å = 12.4 keV (answer).

(b) What is the duration of a cycle in a 1-Å x-ray?
Solution: Duration is the reciprocal of frequency. Therefore, we apply the formula for frequency:

$$\nu = c/\lambda = (3 \times 10^{8}\ \text{m/s})/(1 \times 10^{-10}\ \text{m/cycle}) = 3 \times 10^{18}\ \text{Hz (cyles/s)}$$

Now, the duration: $1/\nu = 3.3 \times 10^{-19}$ s/cycle (duration of one cycle) (answer).

1. The EM Spectrum

Figure 1.9 gives the frequencies, wavelengths, and energies of the various EM radiations. Notice that there are no distinct boundaries among the various types;

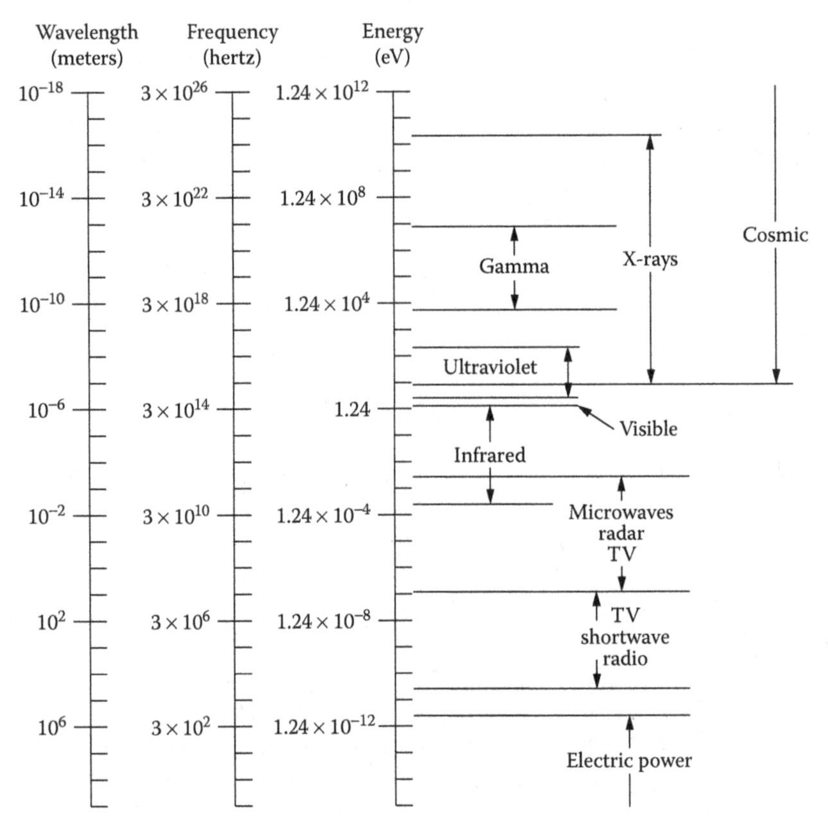

FIGURE 1.9 The EM spectrum. Many regions overlap. Visible light occupies a narrow band in the middle of the spectrum.

some ranges do overlap. For example, x-rays overlap with gamma rays. The difference of course is the origin: x-rays are extra-nuclear; gamma rays are strictly nuclear. Visible light occupies a very narrow band in the middle of the spectrum. Its high-energy side, the violet component, consists of photons carrying 3.1 eV photons and a wavelength of 4,000 Å; the low-energy side, the red component, consists of photons carrying 1.65 eV of energy and having a wavelength of 7,500 Å.

V. PARTICLE INTERACTIONS

A. General Considerations

1. Electrical Charge

Alpha particles, positrons, and negatrons are electrically charged particles. Their interactions depend greatly on their mass, kinetic energy, and the strength of the electrical field they carry as they travel through matter.

2. Momentum

Interactions depend also on the momentum particles carry. A particle's momentum is the product of its mass and its velocity:

$$\text{Momentum} = \text{Mass} \times \text{Velocity}$$

Alpha particles carry a large momentum, because their masses equal 4 Da or 7,294 m_e (electron masses). Negatrons and positrons carry small momenta, because their masses equal 1/1836 Da or 1 m_e only.

3. Impulse

Impulse is defined as the action of a force acting over some time:

$$\text{Impulse} = \text{Force} \times \text{Time}$$

The number of interactions per unit of path length is directly related to the impulse of a particle.

Alpha particles have greater impulses than positrons or negatrons, because they travel at slower speeds and spend much more time in the vicinity of atoms and molecules. In addition, they carry stronger electrical fields. Therefore, they are much more ionizing than beta particles.

B. Alpha Interactions

1. Trajectory

Alpha particles travel through matter in straight lines. This is due to the large momenta they carry. They are not easily deflected from their path (see Figure 6.7).

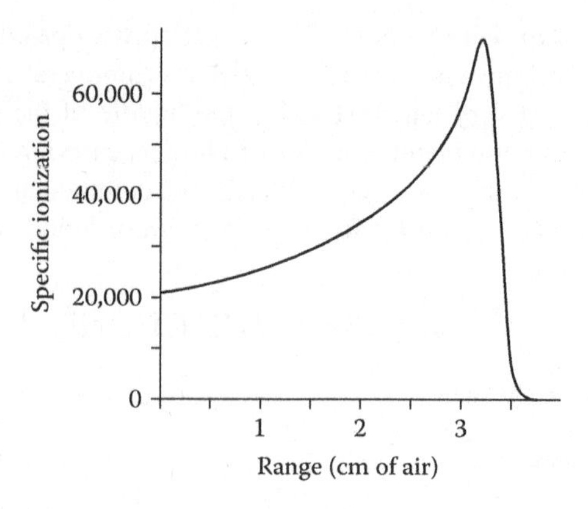

FIGURE 1.10 Bragg curve of polonium-210 alpha particles in air. The specific ionization is plotted against the distance traveled. The energy of the particles is 5.3 MeV and the range in air is 3.6 cm.

2. Range

Their range is short. This is because they are "big spenders" of energy. Their impulses are long and their electrical charge is large. For example, a 5.3-MeV alpha particle of ^{210}Po produces an average of 42,000 ion-pairs/cm in air. At that spending rate, it runs out of energy at 3.6 cm from the point of emission. In soft human tissues, their range is only about 20 μm (see Figure 6.7). Alpha particles are considered high-LET radiations. (LET stands for linear energy transfer; see Chapter 2).

3. Specific Ionization (S)

Specific ionization is the number of ion-pairs produced per centimeter of distance traveled. For electrically charged particles, as in the case of alphas, a graph of specific ionization vs. distance results in a Bragg curve (Figure 1.10): As the particle spends energy by causing ionizations and excitations in matter, it gradually slows down. This, in turn, results in greater impulses. Thus, the specific ionization increases, reaching a maximum just before the particle stops.

C. Beta Interactions (Positrons and Negatrons)

1. Trajectory

Beta particles are easily deflected from their path at each interaction. This is due to their very small momenta. They are said to have a tortuous path.

2. Range

Betas have short impulses. That makes them much less ionizing than alphas. Therefore, they travel much longer distances — about 10 cm to 10 m in air and about 100 μm to 12 mm in soft tissues. Figure 2.3 gives the range of beta particles in any medium.

3. Bremsstrahlung (Braking Radiation)

When a negatron passes near an atomic nucleus, the attractive pull (repulsive force for positrons) of the nucleus slows it down. Under these conditions, a bremsstrahlung photon is emitted. Because the photon is extra-nuclear, it is really an x-ray. This is the way x-rays are produced in radiographic machines.

4. Backscatter

Any beta particle deflected by more than 90° is backscattered. High-Z materials backscatter beta particles more than low-Z materials. Backscatter can be a source of unexpected exposure.

5. Annihilation Radiation

When a positron spends all its energy and comes to a stop, it attracts toward itself a free electron. In an instant, both are converted into two photons of 511-keV each, traveling in opposite directions (180° from each other). Those are the photons detected in PET.

VI. GAMMA RAY INTERACTIONS

A. General Considerations

1. Gamma rays are EM radiations. They have no mass and carry no electrical charge. Yet, they can cause ionizations as they travel through matter.
2. The probability of interaction of a gamma ray is expressed as the apparent cross section of the target. The unit of cross section is the barn (b) = 10^{-24} cm^2.

B. Photoelectric Effect (τ)

1. Photoelectric effect is an interaction of a gamma ray with a tightly bound atomic electron, most likely a K-electron. See Figure 1.11.
2. The gamma ray is completely absorbed and the electron (photoelectron) is ejected (ionization) with a kinetic energy (T) given by

$$T = h\nu - E_b$$

   where $h\nu$ = energy of the gamma ray and E_b = binding energy of the electron.
3. The vacancies in the K-shell and other shells are immediately filled. This results in the emission of characteristic x-rays and/or Auger electrons.
4. Photoelectric effect is more probable with low-energy gamma rays and in high-Z materials:

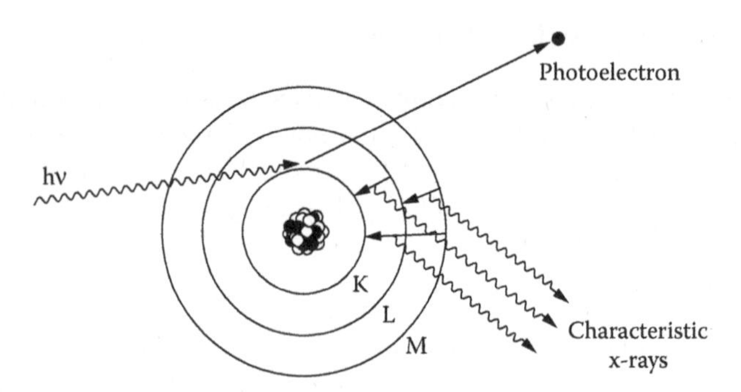

FIGURE 1.11 Photoelectric effect. A gamma ray interacts with a tightly bound electron. The gamma ray is completely absorbed. The electron (photoelectron) is ejected. The rearrangement of electrons that follows results in the emission of a shower of x-rays and/or Auger electrons.

$$\tau = KZ^5/h\nu^{-3}$$

This simply means that the probability of photoelectric effect is directly related to the fifth power of the atomic number of the material and inversely related to the cube of the gamma-ray energy. In NM, lead is the least expensive high-Z material. This makes it the material of choice for shielding against gamma radiation. See also shielding in Chapter 6.

5. The probabilities of photoelectric effect decrease with energy (see Figure 1.15).

C. Compton Effect (σ)

1. Compton effect is an interaction between a gamma ray and a loosely bound or free electron. Figure 1.12 shows a diagram of this interaction.
2. The gamma ray transfers some of its energy to the electron (Compton electron) and is deviated from its original trajectory at any angle.
3. The kinetic energy (T) of the electron is equal to the energy of the original photon minus the energy of the deflected photon:

$$T = h\nu - h\nu'$$

where hν′ = energy of the deflected photon.

4. The probability of Compton interaction is independent of the atomic number of the material and it decreases with the energy of the gamma ray (see Figure 1.15).
5. Arthur Compton demonstrated that the energy of the deflected photon is inversely related to the angle of deflection θ:

$$h\nu' = h\nu/[1 + (h\nu/511)(1 - \cos\theta)]$$

For example, a 662-keV gamma ray of ^{137}Cs, deflected by 30°, would carry 564 keV, and the T of the Compton electron would be 98 keV.

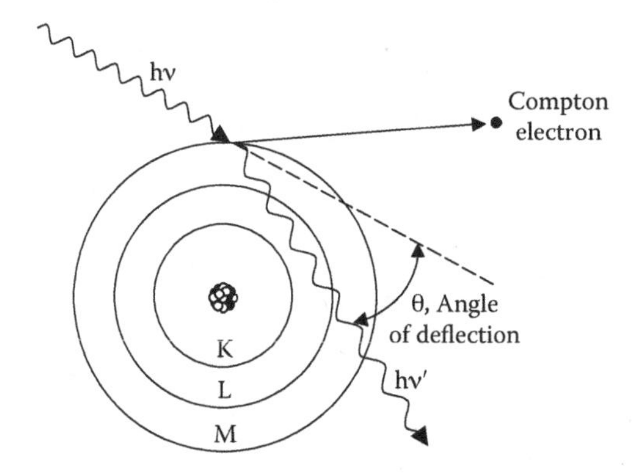

FIGURE 1.12 Compton effect. A gamma ray interacts with a loosely bound electron. The gamma ray is deflected and the electron (Compton electron) is ejected. The energies of both are a function of the angle of deflection.

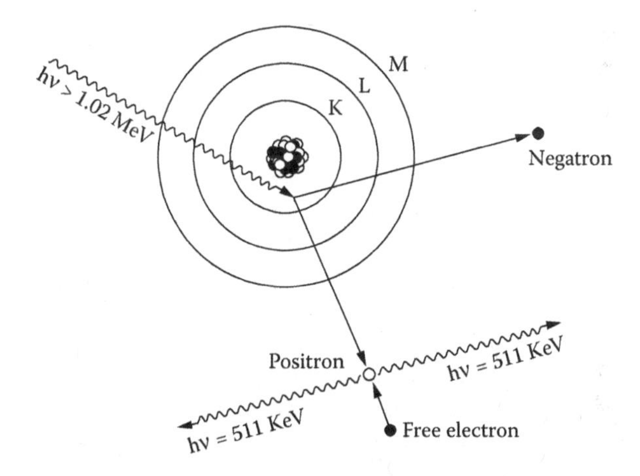

FIGURE 1.13 Pair production. A high-energy gamma ray interacts with the electrical field of an atomic nucleus in a high-Z material and is converted into two electrons: a negatron and a positron. The positron undergoes annihilation radiation.

D. Pair Production (κ)

1. Pair production is an interaction between a gamma ray whose energy is at least 1.02 MeV and the strong electrical field of an atomic nucleus (Figure 1.13).
2. The gamma ray is completely absorbed; 1.02 MeV of the gamma energy is spent in the creation of two electrons, one positively charged and one negatively charged: e^+ and e^-. Any energy above 1.02 MeV is shared by the electrons in the form of kinetic energy. Because the positron is repelled by the nucleus, it usually carries a larger share of the energy.

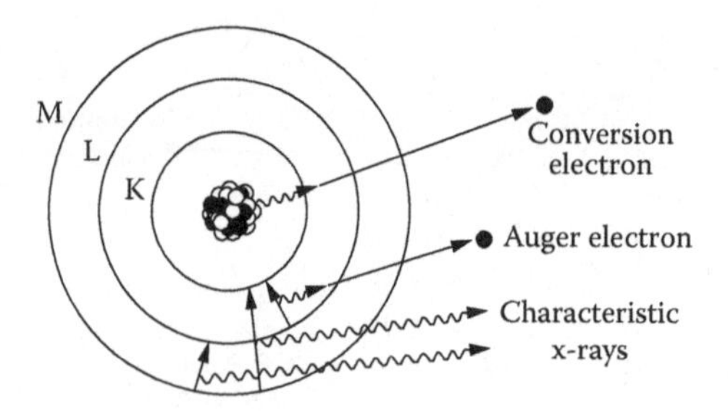

FIGURE 1.14 Internal conversion. A gamma ray interacts with a K electron of the same atom. The gamma ray is absorbed and the electron (conversion electron) is ejected. The rearrangement of electrons that follows results in a shower of x-rays and/or Auger electrons.

3. The positron immediately undergoes annihilation radiation.
4. The probability of pair production increases with energy starting at 1.02 MeV.

E. Internal Conversion (IC)

1. Internal conversion is an interaction of a gamma ray with an orbital electron of the same atom (Figure 1.14).
2. As a result, the gamma ray is completely absorbed, and the orbital electron (conversion electron) is ejected with an energy equal to

$$T = h\nu - E_b$$

   where E_b = binding energy of the electron.
3. Conversion electrons are monoenergetic.
4. This interaction is more likely to occur with the K-electron and less likely to occur with the L- and M-electrons.
5. The vacancies in the various orbitals refill with the emission of characteristic x-rays and/or Auger electrons.

VII. GAMMA RAY INTERACTIONS WITH LEAD AND WATER

A. Some Properties of Lead

1. Atomic number: 82; mass number: 207; density: 11.34 g/cm^3
2. Inexpensive; a heavy metal poison

B. Some Properties of Water

1. Molecular weight: 18; components: hydrogen and oxygen; density: 1 g/cm^3.

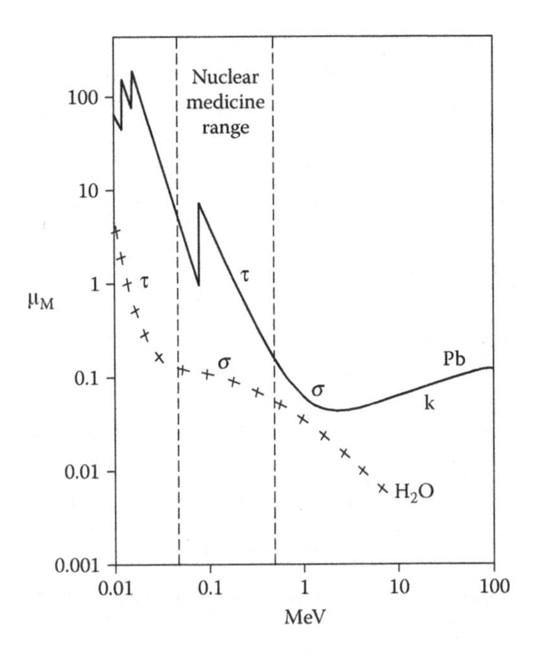

FIGURE 1.15 Probability of gamma ray interactions as a function of energy. Two curves are shown: one for lead, the most important shielding material, and one for water, representing human soft tissues. In the NM range of energies, photoelectric effect predominates in lead and Compton effect predominates in water.

2. Attenuation coefficients of water are almost identical to those of soft tissue.
3. The human body is approximately 2/3 water.
4. Liquid state at human body temperature.

C. Gamma Ray Attenuation

1. The attenuation of a collimated gamma beam is an exponential function of shield thickness. See Chapter 6.
2. The attenuation coefficient is an expression of the probability of attenuation per unit thickness of shield. It also expresses the quality of the shield as an attenuator of gamma rays.
3. Figure 1.15 is a logarithmic graph of the probability of attenuation, expressed as the mass attenuation coefficient on the vertical axis vs. gamma energy in the horizontal axis. The graph shows two curves: one for lead, the most important shielding material, and one for water, representing human soft tissues. Some comments follow.

D. In Lead

1. Photoelectric effect decreases with energy. There are breaks on the curve due to the binding energies of the K-, L-, and M-electrons in lead atoms.

2. At 50 keV, the photoelectric effect is two orders of magnitude (one hundred times) more probable than the Compton effect.
3. Pair production starts at 1.02 MeV and increases with energy.
4. In the range of gamma energies used in NM imaging of about 50 to 511 keV, photoelectric is the most predominant effect in lead. This means complete absorption of the gamma rays, a very desirable effect.

E. In Water or Soft Tissue

1. Compton effect is the predominant one.
2. Compton effect decreases with energy.
3. There is no pair production effect in water.
4. In the range of NM gamma energies, Compton interactions mean minimal absorption and, therefore, low radiation doses to patients and technologists.

PROBLEMS

The problems that follow deal with radioactive decay calculations that occur every day in the practice of NM.

1. A solution of ^{18}F-FDG (fluorodeoxyglucose) has a concentration of 444 MBq/ml at 8:00 a.m. What will the concentration be at 9:14 a.m.?
2. We have a solution of ^{99m}Tc-DTPA whose concentration is 1,258 MBq/ml at noon on Monday. What volume must be drawn for a 925-MBq dosage the same day at 4:00 p.m.?
3. A patient received 7.4 GBq of ^{131}I. The urinary excretion at 24 h was 4.14 GBq. How much radioactivity remains in the patient?
4. A ^{99m}Tc generator arrives on Monday at 8:00 a.m. containing 7.5 GBq of ^{99}Mo. What was its activity at shipping time the previous Friday noon?
5. What are the rates of decay of ^{99}Mo and ^{99m}Tc?
6. The radioactivity of a source decays from 40,000 c/min to 25,000 counts/min in 3 h. What is its half-life?
7. A vial contains 3.7 GBq of ^{99m}Tc-Pertechnetate at 6:00 a.m.. At what time will the activity decay to 2.96 GBq?
8. The activity of a source drops from 50 to 35 MBq in 6.6 h. What is the half-life of the source?
9. What is the activity of 1 billion atoms of ^{99m}Tc?
10. At closing time, 5:00 p.m. Friday, 185 MBq of ^{99m}Tc are spilled in the Hot Lab. What would the activity be at 8:00 a.m. on Monday if no decontamination was done?

REFERENCES

Bethge, K. et al., *Medical Applications of Nuclear Physics*, Springer-Verlag, Berlin, 2004.
Blatner, D., *The Joy of π*, Walker Publishing Company, New York, 1999.

Bouchet, L.G. et al., Consideration in the selection of radiopharmaceuticals for palliation of bone pain from metastatic osseous lesions, *J. Nucl. Med.*, 41, 682, 2000.

Chandra, R., *Nuclear Medicine Physics — The Basics*, 6th ed., Lippincott Williams & Wilkins, Philadelphia, 2004.

Clark, J.O.E., Editor, *The Essential Dictionary of Science*, Barnes & Noble Books, New York, 2004.

De Pree, C.G. and Axelrod, A., Editors, *Van Nostrand's Concise Encyclopedia of Science*, John Wiley & Sons, Hoboken, 2003.

Emiliani, C., *The Scientific Companion*, 2d ed., Wiley Popular Science, New York, 1995.

Hakim, J., *The Story of Science — Aristotle Leads the Way*, Smithsonian Books, Washington, 2004.

Kolestinov-Gautier, H. et al., Evaluation of toxicity and efficacy of ^{186}Re-hydroxyethylidene diphosphonate in patients with painful bone metastases of prostate and breast cancer, *J. Nucl. Med.*, 41, 1689, 2000.

Kowalsky, R.J. and Falen, S.W., *Radiopharmaceuticals in Nuclear Pharmacy and Nuclear Medicine*, 2d ed., American Pharmacists Association, Washington, 2004.

Lederer, C. M., Hollander, J. M., and Perlman, I., *Table of Isotopes*, 6th ed., John Wiley & Sons, New York, 1967.

Lyons, W.A., *The Handy Science Answer Book*, 2d ed., Barnes & Noble Books, New York, 2003.

Maor, E., *e: The Story of a Number*, Princeton University Press, Princeton, 1999.

Pandit-Taskar, N. et al., Radiopharmaceutical therapy for palliation of bone pain from osseous metastases, *J. Nucl. Med.*, 45, 1358, 2004.

Phosphocol® P 32, package insert, Mallinckrodt, St. Louis, 2000.

Rad.Radiological Health Handbook, U.S. Department of Health, Education, and Welfare. Rockville, MD, 1970.

Saha, G.B., *Physics and Radiobiology of Nuclear Medicine*, Springer-Verlag, New York, 1993.

Saha, G.B., *Basics of PET Imaging*, Springer-Verlag, New York, 2005.

Shleien, B., Slaback, Jr., L.A., and Birky, B.K., *Handbook of Health Physics and Radiological Health*, 3d ed., Lippincott Williams & Wilkins, Philadelphia,1998.

Silverstein, E.B. et al., SNM guidelines for palliative therapy of painful bone metastases, in *SNM Proceeding Guidelines Manual, Society of Nuclear Medicine*, Reston, 2003.

Sorenson, J.A. and Phelps, M.E., *Physics in Nuclear Medicine*, 2d ed., W.B. Saunders Company, Philadelphia, 1987.

Statkiewicz-Sherer, M.A., Visconti, P.J., and Ritenour, E.R., *Radiation Protection in Medical Radiography*, 2d ed., Mosby, St. Louis, 1993.

Steves, A.M., *Review of Nuclear Medicine Technology*, 2d ed., Society of Nuclear Medicine, Reston, 1996.

Wagner, H. N. et al., Administration guidelines for radioimmunotherapy of non-Hodgkins lymphoma with ^{90}Y-labeled anti-CD20 monoclonal antibody, *J. Nucl. Med.*, 43, 267, 2002.

Wolfson, R., *Einstein's Relativity and the Quantum Revolution*, 2d ed., The Teaching Company, Chantilly, 2000.

2 Units of Radiation Exposure and Dose

I. RATIONALE

The best weapon against radiation overexposure in the workplace is knowledge. To protect themselves from unnecessary exposure or overexposure, radiation workers must learn as much as possible about the nature, the types, the properties, and the interactions of radiations. They must learn also about the means of protection and the rules and regulations that guarantee their safety and the safety of the general public. To ensure a safe working environment in the NM department, technologists must be able to qualify and quantify radioactivity and radiation fields.

To qualify means to detect the presence of radioactivity, even at very low levels, and to determine its nature, for example, to distinguish beta radiation from gamma radiation. To accomplish this, radiation workers must learn to use survey instruments very well. To quantify radiation means to express in numbers, the quantity of radioactivity or the intensity of a radiation field. To achieve all these goals, they must learn the basic concepts of radioactivity, exposure, and dose and their units. The latter is precisely the objective of this chapter.

II. BASIC CONCEPTS

The five basic concepts that relate a radiation worker to a source of radiation are (1) activity (A), measured in becquerels (Bq) or in curies (Ci); (2) exposure (X), measured in Coulombs/kg of air or in roentgens (R); (3) absorbed dose (D), measured in grays or in rads, (4) equivalent dose (H_T), measured in sieverts or in rems, and (5) effective dose (E), also measured in sieverts or in rems. Figure 2.1 and Table 2.3 show the five concepts and their units.

Note that in many hospitals, clinics, radiopharmacies, and PET centers, the traditional system of units (curie, roentgen, rad, and rem) is still being used in the daily practice of NM. In scientific literature, many articles use both, the international system of units (becquerel, C/kg, gray, and sievert) and the traditional system of units mentioned. For that reason, in this book, both systems are defined and given whenever possible. Appendix C in this book has a table of interconversion of units between the two systems. Readers, NMTs, and NMT students can use it to corroborate their calculations.

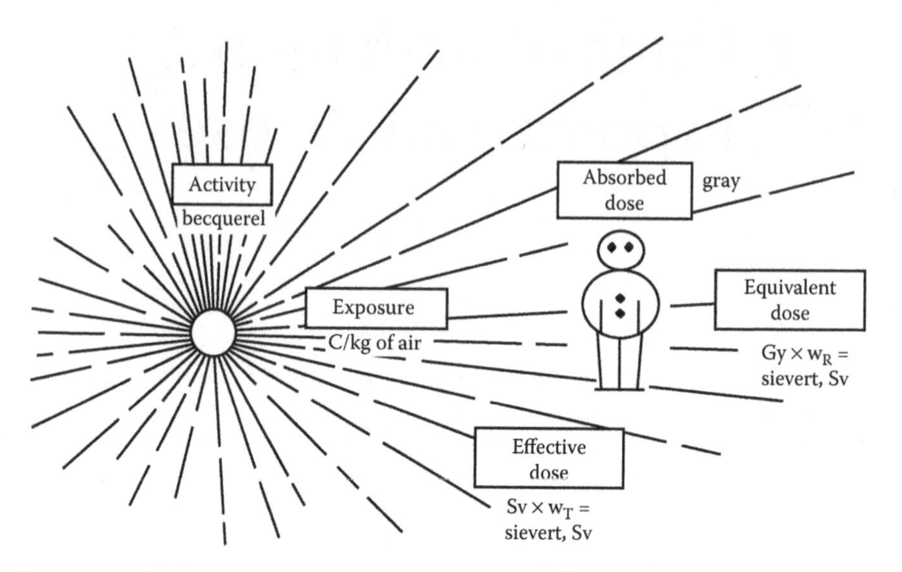

FIGURE 2.1 The five concepts that relate a radiation worker to a radioactive source: Activity, measured in becquerels; Exposure, measured in C/kg of air; Absorbed dose, measured in grays; Equivalent dose, measured in sieverts; and Effective dose, also measured in sieverts.

A. Activity (A)

Activity is an abbreviation of radioactivity. Activity is the number of radioactive atoms (N) decaying per unit time (t). The formal expression is

$$A = N/t \tag{2.1}$$

The S.I. unit of activity is the becquerel (Bq), which is equal to one nuclear transformation per second (1 nt/s). Multiples are kBq = 1000 nt/s, MBq = 1 million (10^6) nt/s, and GBq = 1 billion (10^9) nt/s. The special or traditional units are the curie = 3.7×10^{10} nt/s, with its submultiples mCi = 3.7×10^7 nt/s, and μCi = 3.7×10^4 nt/s.

Quantification (standardization) of a radioactive source can be accomplished by relative and absolute methods of standardization. In NM, the interest lies on gamma emitting radionuclides. The methods are briefly described here.

1. Relative Standardization

The relative method makes use of a standard, a source of certified known activity. Both the standard and the source of unknown activity are measured under the same conditions. Then, the activity of the unknown source is determined using a proportion:

$$\frac{R_x}{R_s} = \frac{A_x}{A_s} \tag{2.2}$$

where R_x = count rate of the unknown source, R_s = count rate of the standard, A_x = activity of the unknown source, and A_s = activity of the standard.

2. Absolute Standardization

The absolute method does not use a standard. The observed count rate of the unknown source is corrected for some well-known physical properties of the radionuclide in question.

The most important properties for gamma emitters are

a. *Gamma fraction*, f_γ, is the fraction of all gamma emissions that corresponds to the main peak of the gamma spectrum. During measurement, the spectrometer window is set to enclose the main peak. Gamma fractions are found in tables along with decay schemes.
b. *Geometry* (G), is the solid angle subtended between a point source and the cylindrical crystal detector at a given distance. This is also the fraction of all gamma emissions that is being intercepted by the crystal detector.
c. *Intrinsic peak efficiency*, E_p, is found in tables for different sizes of crystal detectors. E_p increases with crystal size.

The activity of the unknown (A_x) is then calculated as follows:

$$A_x = \frac{R_x}{F_\gamma \cdot G \cdot E_p} \tag{2.3}$$

In hospitals and clinics, quantification of medical radionuclides is done using well-maintained dose calibrators. See Chapter 4.

B. Exposure (X)

Exposure is the sum of all the electrical charges (Q) of one sign produced by x- or gamma rays in a given mass (m) of dry air at standard temperature and pressure (STP). The formal expression for exposure is

$$X = Q/m \tag{2.4}$$

The S.I. unit of exposure is the Coulomb per kg (C/kg) of dry air at STP. The special unit of exposure is the roentgen (R), defined as 2.58×10^{-4} C/kg of dry air at STP. This definition applies only to x- or gamma rays under 3 MeV of energy. One C/kg is equal to 3876 roentgens.

The intensity of an x- or gamma radiation field is defined as the number of photons passing through a cross section of 1 cm^2 at some distance from the source. This is sometimes referred to as *flux*, and should not be confused with the energy carried by each photon. Intensity is usually measured in terms of exposure rate at some distance from the source, and is usually expressed in milliroentgens per hour (mR/h) or microsieverts/h (μSv/h). The reason for using μSv/h is shown later in this

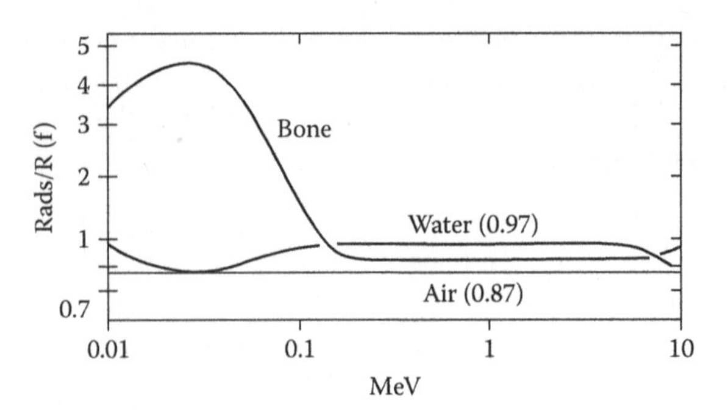

FIGURE 2.2 The f value (rad/R) as a function of gamma ray energy. In the NM range of energies, for most tissues, exposure to 1R of gamma rays results in the absorbed dose of 1 rad.

chapter (Figure 2.2). In water or soft tissue, one roentgen is about equal to one rad, and because the weighting factor for gamma rays is 1, one rad is also equal to one Sv, a unit of equivalent dose. Intensities are measured using calibrated Geiger counters or ionization chambers (Chapter 4). For a point source, the intensity of a radiation field decreases inversely with the square of the distance. This statement is known as the *inverse square law*. Please refer to Chapter 6 for a full description.

C. Absorbed Dose (D)

Absorbed dose (D) is the radiation energy (E) transferred to a unit mass (m) of any material. The formal expression is

$$D = E/m \tag{2.5}$$

The S.I. unit of absorbed dose is the gray (Gy), which is equal to the absorption of one joule of energy per kg of any material including the body of a patient or that of a technologist.

Reminder: In the macroworld, the MKS system (meter, kilogram, second) is used. The unit of energy is the joule. One joule (J) = force of one newton (N) acting over a distance of one meter. One newton = force that gives a mass of 1 kilogram an acceleration of one meter per second each second. Thus, 1 N = 1 kg/s^2 and 1 J = 1 N · m or 1 kg · m/s^2.

The special unit of absorbed dose is the rad (radiation absorbed dose), defined as the absorption of one hundredth of a joule per kg of any material or 1 rad = 0.01 J/kg of material.

To measure the absorbed dose by radiation workers, calibrated dosimeters are used. Examples are film badges and thermoluminescent dosimetry (TLD) badges to monitor body dose, and TLD ring dosimeters to monitor hand dose (Chapter 8).

D. Equivalent Dose ($H_{T,R}$)

This concept replaces the former "dose equivalent," and was introduced to account for the differences in the ionizing quality of the various types of radiations. Equivalent

TABLE 2.1
Radiation Weighting Factors

Radiation	w_R
Beta, gamma, x-rays	1
Neutrons, <10 keV	5
>10-100 keV	10
>100 keV-2 MeV	20
>2 MeV-20 MeV	10
>20 MeV	5
Protons, >2 MeV	2
Alpha, heavy ions	20

dose is defined as the product of the average absorbed dose ($D_{T,R}$) received by tissue ($_T$) from radiation ($_R$) times the radiation weighting factor (w_R):

$$H_{T,R} = D_{T,R} \times w_R \tag{2.6}$$

Average doses, $D_{T,R}$, are expressed in grays (Gy) and equivalent doses, $H_{T,R}$, are expressed in sieverts (Sv). Radiation weighting factors (w_R) recommended by the NCRP are listed in Table 2.1. They replace the former quality factors (Q). The following example illustrates the concept of equivalent dose: A person accidentally inhales some radioactive dust. The absorbed dose to the respiratory tract is 50 mGy from alpha particles, 30 mGy from beta radiation, and 20 mGy from gamma rays. The total absorbed dose is 50 + 30 + 20 = 100 mGy, but the equivalent dose takes into account the quality of each radiation by introducing the radiation weighting factors (w_R). The equivalent dose is

$$(50 \times 20) + (30 \times 1) + (20 \times 1) = 1050 \text{ mSv}$$

E. Effective Dose (E)

Due to the fact that organs and tissues have different sensitivities to radiation, the concept of effective dose (E) was introduced and is defined as the sum of the products of the equivalent doses ($H_{T,R}$) received by an organ times the tissue weighting factors (w_T):

$$E = \Sigma(H_{T,R} \times w_T) \tag{2.7}$$

Effective doses are also expressed in sieverts (Sv). Table 2.2 shows the NRCP-recommended tissue-weighting factors (w_T). An example will illustrate the meaning of w_T: As shown in Table 2.2, an effective dose of 10 mSv to the bone marrow has 12 times the risk of stochastic effect than the same dose to the skin (0.12 vs. 0.01).

TABLE 2.2
Tissue Weighting Factors

Tissue	w_T
Gonads	0.20
Bone marrow	0.12
Colon	0.12
Lung	0.12
Stomach	0.12
Bladder	0.05
Breast	0.05
Liver	0.05
Esophagus	0.05
Thyroid	0.05
Skin	0.01
Bone surface	0.01
Remainder	0.05
Total Body	**1.00**

As an example of "risk," the International Commission on Radiation Protection (ICRP) and the National Council on Radiation Protection (NCRP) have estimated that the risk of fatal cancer for radiation workers is 4×10^{-2} per Sv or 1 cancer per 25 Sv. Technologists receive less than 1% of that dose in 30 years of professional practice. That is very reassuring provided that radiation safety is practiced constantly in the workplace.

F. Relative Biological Effectiveness (RBE)

In radiobiology, the science that studies radiation effects on biological systems, the relative biological effectiveness (RBE) concept is used to account for the sensitivities of different biological systems to alpha radiation, beta radiation, electron beams, neutron fluxes of various energies and, of course, x- and gamma rays. RBE is the ratio of the dose of 250 kVP (kilovolt-peak) x-rays, which produces some effect, to the dose of another radiation that produces the same effect in the same degree. RBEs are useful to radiobiologists when they compare results of experiments done at different locations.

III. OTHER CONCEPTS

A. Specific Ionization

Specific ionization is the number of ion pairs produced by radiation per unit of path length, usually per centimeter of air or per micrometer of soft issue. For example, in air an alpha particle of ^{210}Po, carrying 5.3 MeV of kinetic energy, may produce an average of 42000 ion pairs per cm and stop at 3.6 cm from the point of emission.

B. The W Value

The W value is the average energy required to produce an ion-pair in a medium. In air, W = 33.7 eV; in water, W = 35 eV.

C. Linear Energy Transfer (LET)

LET is defined as the average energy imparted per unit of path length. For x-rays and gamma rays in water and soft tissue, LET is expressed in keV/μm.

D. Range of Beta Particles

Figure 2.3 gives the range of beta particles in any material expressed in density thickness, mg/cm^2. Any value read on the graph can be converted into the corresponding range in water or soft tissues by dividing it by the density of water: 1,000 mg/cm^3.

E. The f Value (rad/R)

For the purpose of discussion, in this case it is preferable to use the classic units of rads per roentgen, also known as the *f value*. When a biological system is placed in an x-ray or gamma ray field whose exposure rate is known, the energy absorbed by that system depends on the energy of the photons and on the nature of the system. Figure 2.2 shows several curves of the f value vs. photon energy. The curves are for air, water (or soft tissue), and for compact bone. Several comments are due regarding the curves:

1. In air, from 10 keV to 10 MeV, the energy dissipation remains constant at 0.87 rad/R.
2. In water or soft tissue, in the range of 150 keV to 5 MeV, energy dissipation remains constant at 0.97 rad/R.
3. In water and soft tissue, below 150 keV, energy dissipation decreases from 0.97 to 0.87 rad/R.
4. In NM, most gamma and x-ray exposures fall in the range of 10 to 511 keV. Therefore, most energy dissipations for NM workers, as well as for patients, fall at 0.97 rad/R or just about 1 rad/R.
5. In compact bone, energy dissipation of photons above 150 keV remains constant at 0.9 rad/R.
6. For bone, below 150 keV, the f value increases inversely with energy from 1 to 4.5 rad/R. This effect is due to the high density of bone.
7. The radiation-sensitive bone marrow is really soft tissue and, therefore, absorbs energy at an f value of about 1 rad/R.
8. Comment: This also means that exposure rates in air in mR/h resemble absorbed dose rates in mrad/h in soft tissues (actually they are lower by 11.5%). Because the radiation weighting factor for gamma rays is 1, they also resemble equivalent dose rates in μSv/h. Table 2.3 is a summary of the basic concepts and their S.I. units.

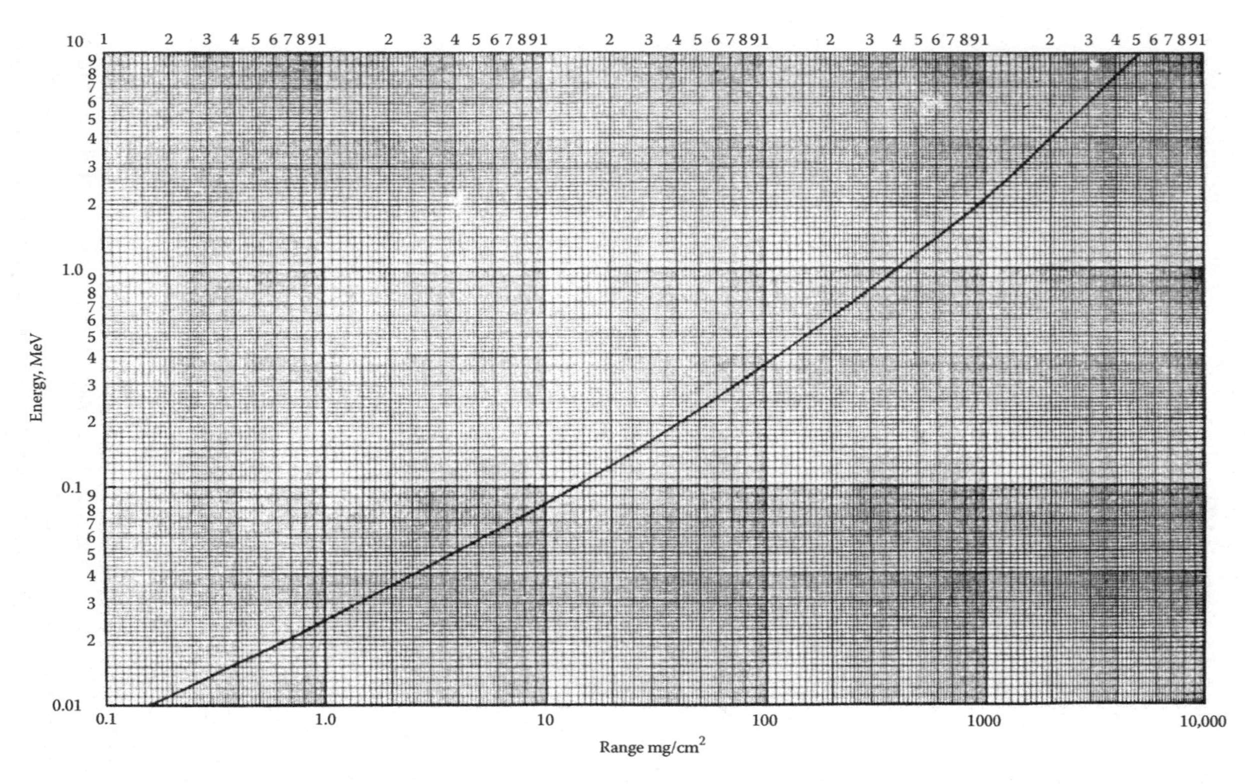

FIGURE 2.3 Range of beta particles in any material. The maximum energy (E_{max}) is plotted against density–thickness. To find the range in water or soft tissues, divide the range found in mg/cm^2 by the density of water, 1000 mg/cm^3.

TABLE 2.3
Summary of Basic Concepts and Units

Concept	Unit and Definition
Activity (A)	becquerel (Bq) = 1 nt/s
	curie (Ci) = 3.7×10^{10} nt/s
Exposure (X)	1 C/kg of air at STP
	roentgen (R) = 2.58×10^{-4} C/kg of air at STP
Absorbed dose (D)	gray (Gy) = 1 J/kg in any material
	rad = 0.01 J/kg of any material
Equivalent dose ($H_{T,R}$)	sievert (Sv) = Gy $\times$ w_R
	rem = rad $\times$ Q
Effective dose (E)	sievert (Sv) = Sv $\times$ w_T
	rem = rad $\times$ w_T

IV. SPECIFIC GAMMA CONSTANT (Γ)

The specific gamma constant, also called the exposure rate constant or simply the gamma constant, is the exposure rate in R/h at 1 cm from a 1-mCi source. Another way of expressing the specific gamma constant using the S.I. system of units is in μSv/h at 1 meter from a 1-GBq gamma source. Table 2.4 gives the specific gamma constants, in both systems of units, for most radionuclides used in NM. The specific gamma constant is extremely useful when we wish to calculate the exposure rate at some distance of any quantity of radioactivity, even before we approach the source. And, knowing how long a task will take, we can calculate the total dose to the hands, to the eyes, to the chest, or to the pelvic region of the person performing the task.

These calculations will allow better planning to minimize exposure, in accordance with the ALARA concept (Chapter 3). Furthermore, the specific gamma constant is essential in the calibration of radiation-survey instruments.

Sample Problems

a. Using Figure 2.3, calculate the maximum range of ^{32}P beta particles in soft tissue.
   Solution: E_{max} for ^{32}P negatrons is 1.71 MeV. The graph gives a range of 800 mg/cm^2. Assuming a density of 1 g/cm^3 for soft tissues, the range in tissues is (800 mg/cm^2)/(1,000 mg/cm^3) = 0.8 cm or 8 mm.
b. What is the expected exposure rate at 50 cm from a 1,750 MBq source of ^{137}Cs?
   Solution: Table 2.4 gives a specific gamma constant of 89.6 μSv/GBq-h at 1 m.

First, 1,750 MBq is equal to 1.75 GBq. Multiplying 89.6 times 1.75 the exposure rate would be 156.8 μSv/h at 1 m. Second, according to the inverse square law, reducing the distance to one-half quadruples the exposure rate. Therefore, 156.8 $\times$

TABLE 2.4
Specific Gamma Constants in Nuclear Medicine

Radionuclide	R/mCi-h at 1 cm	μSv/GBq-h at 1 m
^{51}Cr	0.18	4.9
^{186}Re	0.2	5.4
^{201}Tl	0.46	12.4
^{153}Sm	0.46	12.4
^{133}Xe	0.53	14.3
^{99m}Tc	0.78	21.1
^{57}Co	1.0	27.0
^{125}I	1.43	38.6
^{99}Mo	1.47	39.7
^{123}I	1.63	44.0
^{131}I	2.27	61.3
^{111}In	3.21	86.7
^{137}Cs	3.32	89.6
^{18}F	5.73	154.7
^{11}C	5.91	159.6
^{13}N	5.91	159.6
^{15}O	5.91	159.6
^{68}Ga	6.63	178.9
^{82}Rb	6.1	164.7
^{226}Ra	8.25	222.8
^{60}Co	12.87	347.5

4 = 634.4 μSv/h (answer). This part can be solved also using the inverse square formula (Chapter 6).

V. ABOUT S.I. UNITS

More than 10 years have passed since the S.I. units were introduced to NM. While reviewing the present scientific literature, the use of both systems of units is noticeable. To expedite full conversion into the S.I. system, the following tasks are recommended:

1. Prescriptions of RPs for patients could be done in rounded MBq only.
2. RP companies could indicate RP concentrations on their vial labels in MBq/ml only.
3. RP package inserts can convert RP dosimetry data to μSv/MBq.
4. NMTs can easily correct for decay in the usual manner. They can calculate volumes needed for patients' dosages in the usual manner.
5. Manufacturers can convert the scales of their survey instruments to read μSv/h, mSv/h, and Sv/h. Manufacturers of dose calibrators can convert their scales to read kBq, MBq, and GBq.

6. Dosimetry companies could submit their personnel dose reports in μSv/month.
7. MDs and other scientists doing clinical and/or basic research could report their results in S.I. units only.

For those who prefer the special units, Appendix C in this book can provide assistance with the interconversion of units between the two systems.

PROBLEMS

1. P-32 beta particles have a maximum range of 800 mg/cm^2 in any material. What is the maximum range in soft tissues?
2. Y-90 beta particles have an E_{max} of 2.38 MeV and a maximum range of 1.22 g/cm^2 in any material. What is their maximum range in soft tissues?
3. What is the dose rate at 30 cm from a 2-MBq source of ^{226}Ra?
4. In an accident, a person receives 100 mGy of 50-keV neutrons and 20 mGy of gamma rays. Calculate the total equivalent dose.
5. What are the S.I. specific gamma constants of ^{123}I, ^{131}I, ^{111}In, and ^{99m}Tc?
6. What are the S.I. gamma constants of ^{18}F, ^{13}N, ^{11}C, and ^{82}Rb?
7. What are the $\bar{E}_\beta$ of ^{32}P, ^{89}Sr, ^{186}Re, and ^{90}Y?
8. What are the $\bar{E}_\beta$ of ^{18}F, ^{13}N, ^{11}C, and ^{82}Rb?
9. What is the dose rate at 1.5 m from a vial containing 500 MBq of ^{18}F-FDG?
10. What is the dose rate at 10 inches from the same vial of Problem 9?

REFERENCES

Bethge, K. et al., *Medical Applications of Nuclear Physics*, Springer–Verlag, Berlin, 2004.

Bevalacqua, J.J., *Basic Health Physics — Problems and Solutions*, Wiley–VCH, Weinheim, 1999.

Chandra, R., *Nuclear Medicine Physics — The Basics*, 6th ed., Lippincott Williams & Wilkins, Philadelphia, 2004.

Chilton, H.M. and Witcofski, R.L., *Nuclear Pharmacy*, Lea & Febiger, Philadelphia, 1986.

Dowd, S.B. and Tilson, E.R., *Practical Radiation Protection and Applied Radiobiology*, 2d ed., Saunders, Philadelphia, 1999.

Indium In-111 Chloride Sterile Solution, package insert, Mallinckrodt, Inc., St. Louis, 2002.

Kowalsky, R.J. and Falen, S.W., *Radiopharmaceuticals in Nuclear Pharmacy and Nuclear Medicine*, 2d ed., American Pharmacists Association, Washington, 2004.

Lederer, C.M., Hollander, J.M., and Perlman, I., *Table of Isotopes*, 6th ed., John Wiley & Sons, New York, 1967.

Noz, M.E, and Maguire, G.Q., *Radiation Protection in the Radiologic and Health Sciences*, 2d ed., Lea & Febiger, Philadelphia, 1985.

Radiological Health Handbook, U.S. Dept. of Health, Education, and Welfare, Rockville, MD, 1970.

Saha, G.B., *Physics and Radiobiology of Nuclear Medicine*, Springer–Verlag, New York,1993.

Sandler, M.P. et al. Editors, *Diagnostic Nuclear Medicine*, Lippincott Williams & Wilkins, Philadelphia, 2003.

Shani, G., *Radiation Dosimetry — Instrumentation and Methods*, 2d ed., CRC Press, Boca Raton, 2000.

Sorenson J.A., and Phelps, M.E., *Physics in Nuclear Medicine*, 2d ed., W.B. Saunders, New York, 1987.

Statkiewicz-Sherer, M.A., Visconti, P.J., and Ritenour, E.R., *Radiation Protection in Medical Radiography*, 2d ed., Mosby, St. Louis, 1993.

Turner, J.E., Editor, *Atoms, Radiation, and Radiation Protection*, 2d ed., John Wiley & Sons, Inc., New York, 1995.

Shleien, B., Slaback, Jr., L.A., and Birky, B.K., *Handbook of Health Physics and Radiological Health*, 3d ed., Lippincott Williams & Wilkins, Philadelphia, 1998.

3 Guidelines for Radiation Protection

I. RATIONALE

Wilhelm Roentgen discovered x-rays in 1895, and Henri Becquerel discovered natural radioactivity in 1896. Marie and Pierre Curie discovered radium and polonium in 1898. Anderson discovered the positron in 1932, and two years later, Frederic and Irene Curie discovered artificial radioactivity. The same year, Lawrence invented the cyclotron. Those events marked the beginning of radiology and nuclear medicine (NM), two specialties that, at present, lend mankind invaluable service in the alleviation of many illnesses. As the nature and properties of those ionizing radiations were unknown in the early days, many persons were injured while working with x-ray machines and handling radioactive materials.

As soon as radiation injuries were recognized, scientists worked diligently to attain a better understanding of the nature, properties, and interactions of ionizing radiations with living and nonliving matter. Those scientists, working in close cooperation with national and international scientific organizations, have made recommendations for the safety of workers and members of the general public. In each country, those recommendations have been translated into laws and regulations aimed at ensuring the safety of individuals and populations.

This chapter presents a description of the agencies responsible for making recommendations, for defining concepts and units of measurement, and for setting radiation safety standards. The concepts and the standards are presented and discussed. Where appropriate, reference is made of the pertinent Code of Federal Regulations (CFR). Finally, an explanation is given on how those standards and regulations are applied in hospitals and clinics.

II. NATIONAL AND INTERNATIONAL AGENCIES

A. The Big Picture

National and international organizations are constantly working to assess the risks and the benefits of radiation in science, medicine, and industry. In the United States, their recommendations are translated into laws by the legislative authorities and then, in the form of regulations, enforced by the Nuclear Regulatory Commission (NRC) or the agreement states' agencies. Figure 3.1 shows diagrammatically the interconnections among those organizations, the NRC, the agreement

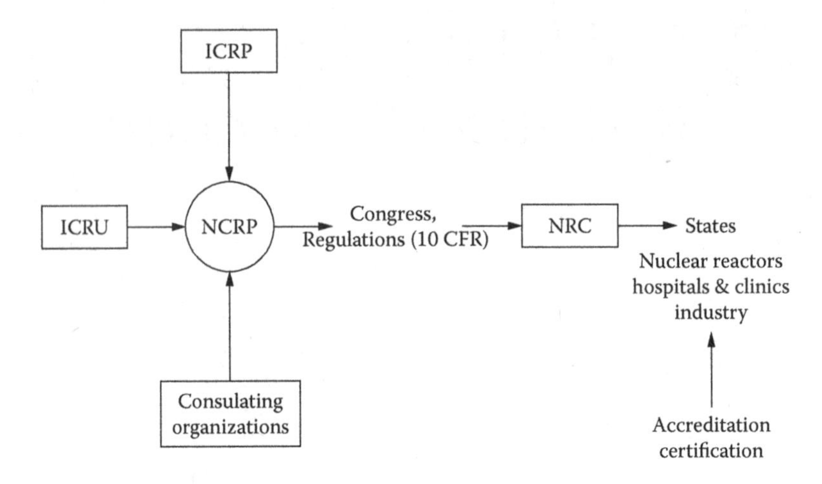

FIGURE 3.1 The big picture: international and national organizations interact with each other in the process of studying and analyzing scientific data and formulating recommendations, standards, rules, and regulations for radiation safety.

states' agencies and the licensees: colleges, universities, government contractors, nuclear power plants, radiopharmaceutical companies, hospitals, clinics, and private industries. Professionals working in those institutions must demonstrate qualifications, engage in continuing education to maintain accreditation, and must periodically renew their licenses during their careers.

B. National Council on Radiation Protection and Measurement

The NCRP is the U.S. agency responsible for studying and analyzing all scientific and technical data regarding ionizing radiations and for making recommendations concerning safety: development, evaluation, and application of basic radiation concepts, measurements, and units. Their recommendations seek maximization of benefits while minimizing the risks of stochastic effects. The council is a nonprofit organization consisting of about 75 members divided into committees. They maintain close communication with many international and national agencies, including the International Commission on Radiation Protection (ICRP), the International Commission on Radiation Units and Measurements (ICRU), the International Atomic Energy Agency (IAEA), the National Academy of Sciences (NAS), the National Science Foundation (NSF), the Radiological Society of North America (RSNA), the Society of Nuclear Medicine (SNM), the Environmental Protection Agency (EPA), the Food and Drug Administration (FDA), and the Department of Transportation (DOT).

C. International Commission on Radiation Protection (ICRP)

The ICRP consists of about 100 members from many countries. Divided into committees, its main objectives are to recommend policies regarding prevention of deterministic effects and limitation of the risk of stochastic effects. Some of the latter are as follows: the linear nonthreshold relationship between the probability of effects and radiation dose at very low levels, the genetic susceptibility to radiation-induced cancer, the role of contaminated lands, and the problem of radiation waste management and disposal, among others. They also define new concepts, standards for radiation safety, and recommend radiation dose limits for workers and for the general public.

D. International Commission on Radiation Units and Measurements

Founded in 1925, the ICRU comprises 19 committees. Its main objective is to make assessments of radiations and their safe and effective use. From those assessments, the commission makes recommendations about definitions of concepts, units, and operations. It is in constant consultation with many agencies. Among them, the following can be mentioned: the United Nations Food and Agricultural Organization (FAO), the International Atomic Energy Agency (IAEA), the United Nations Scientific Committee on the Effects of Atomic Radiation (UNSCEAR), and the World Health Organization (WHO).

E. Nuclear Regulatory Commission (NRC)

The NRC is the agency that enforces the radiation safety laws in the United States. The NRC abides by Title 10 of the Code of Federal Regulations (10CFR) when writing its own regulations, which are distributed among all users of ionizing radiations in approximately 18 states. The other 32 states are "agreement states," which means that they have signed an agreement with the NRC to manage their own radiation safety programs. To do so, they must demonstrate that they have the manpower and resources to take up the task of management and regulation. In so doing, they abide by the NRC regulations. For example, in the state of Florida, which is an agreement state, the Department of Health and Rehabilitative Services (HRS) is the agency responsible for licensing users and enforcing radiation safety laws. In addition, the Agency for Health Care Administration (AHCA) is responsible for safety in laboratories performing *in vitro* radioassays.

F. Environmental Protection Agency (EPA)

The EPA is the U.S. agency responsible for ensuring the good quality of the air and water by setting standards for releases of physical and chemical wastes from industries. The EPA issues regulations under Title 40 of the Code of Federal Regulations (40CFR). Along with the U.S. Centers for Disease Control (CDC), the EPA also makes recommendations on permissible concentrations of radon gases and other radionuclides. See Chapter 7.

G. Food and Drug Administration (FDA)

In addition to approving nonradioactive drugs, the FDA is responsible for the approval of new radiopharmaceuticals (RPs). To gain approval, a diagnostic investigational new drug (IND) must demonstrate through preclinical and clinical trials that it is both safe and effective:

1. *Safe* means that it is neither chemically toxic nor radiotoxic. RPs are considered safe if each dosage does not exceed (a) 3 rem (30 mSv) to the whole body, the bone marrow, the lenses of the eyes, and the gonads, (b) 5 rem (50 mSv) to other organs, and (c) 15 rem (150 mSv) of annual committed equivalent dose.
2. *Effective* means that the RP, in a diagnostic procedure, is both sensitive and specific:
   a. *Sensitivity* is the ability to detect illness, i.e., a high percentage of true positives among all ill patients studied.
   b. *Specificity* is the ability to recognize the healthy state, i.e., a high percentage of true negatives among all healthy volunteers studied.

To expedite the approval of PET RPs, the US Congress passed FDAMA, the FDA Modernization Act, in 2000 by which they streamlined the steps needed for approval.

H. Department of Transportation (DOT)

The DOT is the agency responsible for setting standards for proper packaging, labeling, and transportation of radioactive materials, including radioactive wastes. DOT regulations regarding the transportation of radioactive materials are contained in Title 49 of the CFR. In NM, three categories of radioactive packages are recognized depending on the dose rate at the surface and at a 1-m distance. Table 3.1 gives the maximum dose rates allowed. Figure 3.2 shows the three category labels. All have the radiation symbol. The category I label (lowest level) is white. Labels for categories II and III are yellow and show a "transportation index" (TI), which is the actual dose rate at one meter at the time of shipment. The maximum TI for passenger aircraft transportation is 3 mR/h (30 μSv/h). Shipment of nuclide generators (category III) must abide by that TI. For other industries that ship radioactive materials by cargo airplanes, the TI is 10 mR/h (100 μSv/h). After use, nuclide generators are allowed

TABLE 3.1
Nuclear Medicine Packages

	On the Surface mrem/h (μSv/h)	At 1 m mrem/h (μSv/h)
Category I	0.5 (5)	Background
Category II	50 (500)	1 (10)
Category III[a]	100 (1,000)	3 (30)

[a] Other industries, for packages transported on cargo airplanes the limits are: on the surface: 200 mrem/h (2 mSv/h) and at 1 m: 10 mrem/h (100 μSv/h).

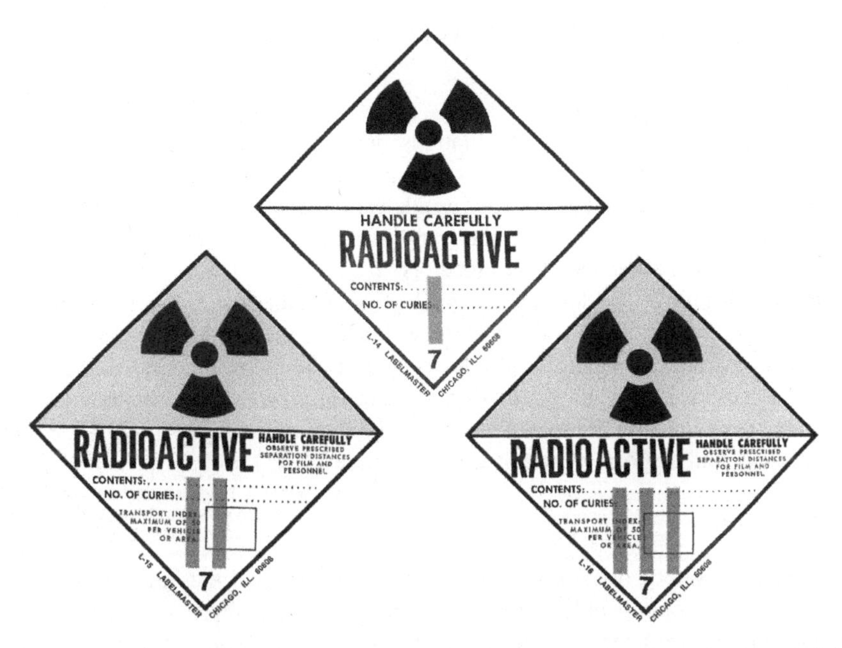

FIGURE 3.2 Labels authorized by the Department of Transportation for packages containing medical radiopharmaceuticals. For categories II and III, the top of each label has a yellow background.

to decay and then, as per manufacturer's instructions, are shipped back for recycling. At this time, the dose rate on the surface of the package must not exceed 0.5 mR/h (5 μSv/h). For international transportation of radioactive materials, the International Atomic Energy Agency (IAEA) guidance should be consulted.

I. Joint Commission on Accreditation of Health Organizations

The JCAHO is the agency responsible for insuring the correct and safe operation of hospitals, clinics, and health organizations. On a regular basis, JCAHO inspects hospitals and clinics. Passing inspection means renewal of accreditation.

J. Other Consulting Organizations

In addition to those organizations mentioned here, the following U.S. organizations are actively involved in the process of establishing safety guidelines: the American Nuclear Society (ANS), the American Medical Association (AMA), the Department of Energy (DOE), the American College of Radiology (ACR), the Society of Nuclear Medicine (SNM), the National Academy of Sciences–Biological Effects of Ionizing Radiation (NAS-BEIR), the National Science Foundation (NSF), the National Institutes of Health (NIH), the National Bureau of Standards (NBS), the Health Physics Society (HPS), and the Occupational Safety and Health Administration (OSHA), among others.

III. RADIATION SAFETY AND THE LAW

A. Objective

The safety of individuals and populations depends on the safe management of radioactive materials and ionizing radiation-producing devices. Radioactive materials include "byproduct materials" such as nuclear fuels (uranium-235 and plutonium-239), their fission fragments, and their products of decay encountered in research nuclear reactors and nuclear power reactors.

Radiation-producing devices are medical and industrial x-ray machines and radioisotopic sources such as cobalt-60, cesium-137, radium-226, plutonium-beryllium, and americium-241, used in industry and in college education. Medical radionuclides include byproduct materials and accelerator-produced radionuclides. NM safety involves the safe management of the production, transportation, possession, use, storage, and disposal of medical radionuclides.

B. Philosophy

For maximum safety, dose limits for radiation workers and the general public are based on the "nonthreshold, linear dose–effect relationship," a hypothesis that assumes that all exposures, no matter how low, do cause some deleterious effect. That assertion may be true for some low-level, long-term (stochastic) effects, but this is still extremely difficult to prove. However, most experts agree that, at this time, it is safe to accept the hypothesis when setting dose limits for radiation workers and the general public. Figure 3.3, curve A, shows the expected percent increase in genetic mutations in humans as a function of radiation dose, which is an example of the nonthreshold, linear dose–effect hypothesis. Figure 3.3, curve B, shows the percentage of persons who become ill after an acute whole-body exposure to a given dose of x- or gamma rays. The latter is an example of a threshold nonlinear relationship (deterministic effect). For a mathematical description of these hypotheses, see Chapter 10.

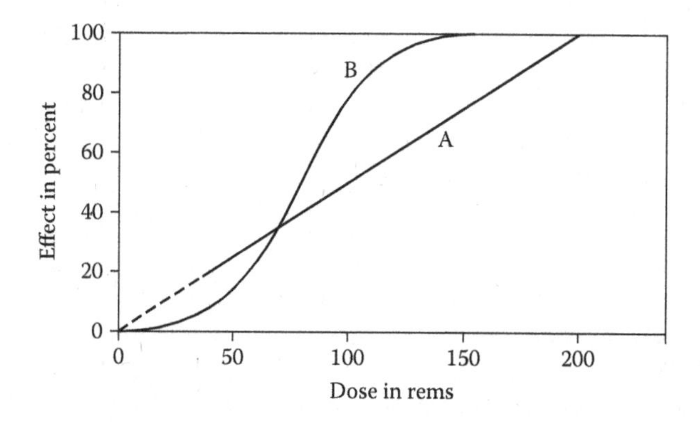

FIGURE 3.3 (A) Stochastic effects: The probability of observing spontaneous mutations increases linearly with radiation dose. (B) Deterministic effects: After a threshold, the severity of radiation illness increases nonlinearly with radiation dose.

C. The Concept of Risk

To deal with stochastic effects in a more realistic way, the NCRP proposed in 1987 that the concept of risk be introduced when evaluating safety in the nuclear industry, as is done in many other industries. In doing so, the assumption was made that the risk of stochastic effect after exposure to low levels of ionizing radiation follows the nonthreshold, linear dose–effect relationship. The use of such radiations was recognized as acceptable because the benefits outweighed the risks. Also stated was that, to reduce the probability of stochastic effects, the policy of ALARA (as low as reasonably achievable) must be implemented in industries using ionizing radiations. For the public, any unnecessary exposure represents an unacceptable risk, because it does not provide any benefit. For patients, the risk of an NM procedure is considered acceptable because the procedure does provide a benefit in terms of diagnostic value followed by the potential for a successful treatment of a properly diagnosed illness. More on risks in Chapter 10.

D. The ALARA Policy

The ALARA policy (10CFR20.1105) was proposed to compensate for the set dose limits. For example, the whole-body dose limit for radiation workers, external exposure, is 5 rem/y (50 mSv/y). That limit seems to imply that 5 rem (50 mSv) is the threshold below which workers are presumed to be safe and contradicts the nonthreshold linear dose–effect hypothesis for stochastic effects. To compensate for that apparent contradiction, the practice of ALARA was recommended in the mid-1980s. In 1994, the NRC made it mandatory. All users must prepare, practice, and revise yearly an ALARA program. In NM practice, all persons must minimize their radiation exposures and that of their co-workers by practicing ALARA at all times. There are two recommended ALARA levels: level I, exceeding 10% of the dose limit (warning level), and level II, exceeding 30% of the dose limit (action level). These rules apply also to releases of radioactivities into effluents (e.g., smoke stacks and sewage systems) and into unrestricted areas.

In each institution using ionizing radiations, the radiation safety officer (RSO) is responsible for enforcing the ALARA program.

E. Method

The safe management of radioactive materials and radiation-producing devices is mandated by state and federal laws. Federal laws are translated into regulations that are published by the Office of the Federal Register National Archives and Records under one or more titles of the Code of Federal Regulations (CFR). The parts pertaining to NM are mainly contained in Title 10:

Part 19: Notices, Instructions, and Reports to Workers: Inspections and Investigations (10CFR19).
Part 20: Standards for Protection against Radiation (10CFR20).
Part 30: Rules Applicable to Licensing of Byproduct Material (10CFR30).
Part 35: Medical Use of Byproduct Materials (10CFR35).

Note: Byproduct material means nuclear fuels such as uranium-235 and plutonium-239, their fission fragments, and products of their radioactive decay.

F. Licensing (10CFR19.3)

The management of byproduct materials must be in the hands of qualified persons and institutions. Radiation workers must demonstrate their qualifications, training, and experience by passing a national certification exam. The NRC, or the applicable state agency in an agreement state, issues licenses to qualified persons and medical institutions. Frequent inspections by those agencies ensure continuing compliance with the terms of the license and renewal as scheduled. In addition, nuclear physicians (NMDs), radiopharmacists (RPs), and nuclear medicine technologists (NMTs) must document their continuing education to maintain accreditation and to renew their licenses.

1. General Licenses

General licenses are issued to physicians, technologists, and clinical laboratories for radiotracer, low-level procedures (nonimaging procedures) such as thyroid uptake of ^{131}I, blood volume measurements, vitamin B_{12} absorption studies, and radioimmunoassays.

2. Specific Licenses

a. *Limited scope*: Issued to physicians and clinics to perform some specific diagnostic or therapeutic NM procedures listed in the license.
b. *Broad scope*: Issued to large hospitals and clinics to perform a broad spectrum of NM procedures and to develop new procedures through research. A radiation safety committee is required. The radiation safety officer (RSO) is responsible for enforcing safety.

IV. TYPES OF RADIATION EFFECTS

A. Acute and Chronic Exposures

Radiation effects depend on the type of exposure. Acute exposure means a high dose delivered within a short time: many rems (mSv to Sv) delivered within seconds to minutes. That type of exposure may be seen in partial-body irradiation during cancer therapy. The results of such exposure are deterministic effects. Chronic exposure means that one or more very low doses are delivered during a long time interval, for example, the exposure received by radiologists and NM personnel in the practice of their professions. The results of this type of exposure are stochastic effects.

B. Deterministic Effects

Deterministic effects are the result of a high-level exposure such as the ones that occur in a radiation accident. In that case, the severity of the effect (injuries, symptoms, and signs of illness) increases with the magnitude of the dose received. Typically, the curve has a threshold below which the effect is not observed. Figure 3.3, curve B, shows that, below 20 rems (200 mSv) of whole-body irradiation with hard x-rays or gamma rays, the signs or symptoms of illness are not observed. This is the threshold for radiation illness. At a dose above 20 rems (200 mSv), the illness, also known as the *acute radiation syndrome* (ARS), becomes more severe, and the severity increases with dose. At a dose of 100 rems (1 Sv), illness approaches 100%, which is the threshold for radiation deaths — another example of deterministic effects. To prevent deterministic effects, such as radiation accidents, experts must set dose limits well below thresholds, and medical personnel must practice radiation safety at all times.

C. Stochastic Effects

In stochastic effects, the probability of observing the effect increases with the dose received. The accepted point of view is that the curve has no threshold and shows that the effect increases linearly with dose. Figure 3.3, curve A, shows the straight-line characteristic of stochastic effects.

In this case, there is an increase in the number of genetic mutations with dose, according to estimates by experts. Notice that the low side of the curve is represented by an interrupted line to indicate that the data are either incomplete or inconclusive. Other examples of stochastic effects are the risk of cancer or leukemia and life shortening. To prevent the risk of stochastic effects, ALARA must be practiced at all times.

V. OTHER CONCEPTS IN DOSIMETRY

The concepts of absorbed dose, equivalent dose, and effective dose were defined in Chapter 2. They represent radiation doses received from external exposure to ionizing radiation. Other important concepts are described next (10CFR20.1003).

A. Committed Equivalent Dose, $H_T(\tau)$

The committed equivalent dose is defined as the total equivalent dose received by the organs or tissues of a radiation worker during the 50 years after the accidental intake of radioactivity. It is measured in rems or Sv, and it is determined at the time of the intake using bioassay procedures. For members of the public, the time is 70 years (an average lifetime).

B. Committed Effective Dose, $E(\tau)$

Committed effective dose is the sum of the products of committed equivalent doses times the tissue weighting factors (w_T):

$$E(\tau) = \Sigma[H_T(\tau) \times w_T] \qquad (3.1)$$

This concept replaces the former committed effective dose equivalent.

TABLE 3.2
Some ALIs and DACs in Nuclear Medicine

Radionuclide	ALIs (μCi) Ingestion	ALIs (μCi) Inhalation	DACs (μCi/ml)
^{133}Xe[a]	—	—	1×10^{-4}
^{131}I, thyroid	30	50	2×10^{-8}
^{131}I, whole body	90	200	—
^{125}I	40	60	3×10^{-6}

[a] Internal dose is negligible.

C. Annual Limit on Intake (ALI)

The annual limit on intake (ALI) is the quantity of a radionuclide, taken by ingestion or inhalation, that results in a committed equivalent dose of 5 rem/y (50 mSv/y) to the whole body or 50 rem/y (500 mSv/y) to any organ. ALIs are measured in microcuries (μCi) or kilobecquerels (kBq). To arrive at committed equivalent doses, radionuclides that enter the body by inhalation are classified in relation to their lung clearance half-times as follows:

1. Class D (days): Have a lung-clearance half-time measured in days.
2. Class W (weeks): Have a lung-clearance half-time measure in weeks.
3. Class Y (years): Have a lung clearance half-time measured in years.

D. Derived Air Concentrations (DACs)

Derived air concentrations (DACs) are concentrations that result in one ALI when a worker is exposed to inhalation or ingestion of radioactivity over one year of light work (2,000 h). DACs are measured in μCi/ml (kBq/ml) of air or water. For medical radionuclides most likely to result in internal contamination, ALIs and DACs are given in Table 3.2.

E. Deep Dose (H_d)

Deep dose is the whole-body dose received at 1 cm depth from external exposure to penetrating radiation (x-rays, gamma rays, and neutrons). This includes all internal organs except the skin and the lenses of the eyes. The deep doses are usually calculated from film or TLD badge readings or other personnel dosimeter readings.

F. Shallow Dose (H_s)

Shallow dose is the dose received by the whole body skin at 70 μm depth, mostly from low penetrating radiations (negatrons, positrons, low-energy photons). The shallow dose is usually divided into H_s-whole body (calculated from TLD or film badge readings) and H_s-extremities (usually calculated from TLD ring dosimeter readings).

G. Lens Dose (LD)

The lens dose is the external dose received at 3-mm depth into the eyes, where the lenses are located. LD is usually calculated from TLD or film badge readings.

VI. RECOMMENDED DOSE LIMITS

Dose limits take into consideration the risk of injury due to accidental acute exposure to high levels of ionizing radiations (deterministic effects) and the risk of injury due to low-level chronic exposure (stochastic effects). The NCRP recommends dose limits for radiation workers and for the general public in their Report 116, 1993. Occupational limits exclude exposures for medical reasons. Limits for the public are usually 10% of those for radiation workers.

A. Occupational Dose Limits (10CFR20.1201)

1. Whole-body, effective equivalent dose	5 rem/y	(50 mSv/y)
2. Cumulative whole-body dose	1 rem × age	(10 mSv × age)
3. Lens of the eye (3-mm deep)	15 rem/y	(150 mSv/y)
4. Skin, hands, and feet	50 rem/y	(500 mSv/y)
5. Declared pregnancy (embryo, fetus)	50 mrem/month	(500 μSv/month)

B. General Public Dose Limits (10CFR20.1301)

1. Whole-body (continuous exposure)	100 mrem/y	(1 mSv/y)
2. Whole-body (infrequent exposure)	500 mrem/y	(5 mSv/y)
3. Lens of the eye	1.5 rem/y	(15 mSv/y)
4. Skin, hands, and feet	5 rem/y	(50 mSv/y)
5. Minors in training, younger than 18	10% of occupational dose limits	

C. Comments

1. In unrestricted areas of NM facilities with accessibility to the public (reception, waiting rooms), the dose limit is 2 mrem/h (20 μSv/h).
2. NM procedures in women of childbearing age: approval of physician; a pregnancy test may be required. Women breast-feeding a child: approval of physician.
3. Exposure to radon gases and their products of decay: According to the NCRP, long-term monitoring resulting in an average concentration of more than 8 pCi per liter of air (0.3 Bq/l of air) requires remedial action. The EPA recommends remedial action at 4 pCi/l of air.
4. Negligible dose: The NCRP has concluded that 1 mrem (10 μSv) is a negligible dose.

VII. RADIATION SAFETY PRACTICE

To complete the picture, a brief outline of how the rules and regulations are applied in the NM departments of hospitals and clinics is given here. A detailed description of radiation safety in the NM department of a large institution is presented in Chapter 5.

A. Radiation Safety Officer (RSO)

The RSO is someone who, by qualifications and experience, is capable of performing, enforcing, and maintaining a radiation safety program in a medical institution (10CFR35.2). Proof of qualifications and experience must be submitted to the licensing agency. The RSO is a person selected by the management of the institution. Usually a physician, a medical physicist, a health physicist, a radiopharmacist, or an NMT can serve as an RSO.

B. Radiation Safety Committee (RSC)

The radiation safety committee is a group of members of the licensed medical institution that oversees the operation of the radiation safety program. Members are the RSO, a nursing representative, a member of the administration (management), and one or more "users." Users are nuclear physicians and nuclear pharmacists. Their names appear in the license. They supervise NMTs and research assistants. The RSC approves changes in the radiation safety program within the confinements of the license.

C. Radiation Safety Program (RSP)

The RSP, also referred to as the radiation protection program (RPP), is a document consisting of internal rules prepared by the RSO and adopted by the RSC. The program reflects the terms of the license under the type of operation of the hospital or clinic. Revisions to the program are made once a year (10CFR20.1105).

D. Quality Management Program (QMP)

The QMP is a document submitted to the licensing agency by the licensee giving a detailed description of the procedure for prescribing, preparing, dispensing, administering, and recording dosages of radiopharmaceuticals. The objective is to prevent misadministration of radioactive drugs to patients. The QMP must include methods of reporting, documenting, and recording misadministration. The QMP is revised once a year. See also Chapter 5.

E. The ALARA Program

The ALARA program is a document submitted by the licensee to the licensing agency that gives methods for providing the staff with information and training on radiation safety matters, on radiation dose limits, on means to reduce personnel exposures, and on continuing education (10CFR20.1105). The program may include

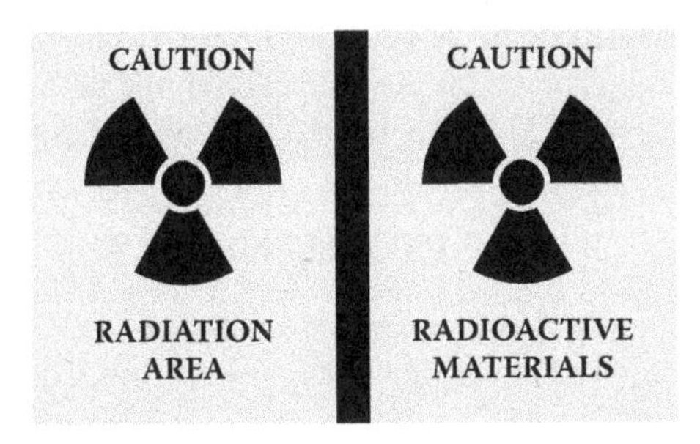

FIGURE 3.4 Two radiation warning signs. Symbols are printed in magenta over a yellow background.

policies regarding pregnant workers, storage of radioactive sources, and other issues that may be specific to the institution. The ALARA program may be included in the radiation safety program.

F. Radiation Warning Signs

The RSO is responsible for placing radiation warning signs on locations prescribed by the levels of radioactivity, certain exposure rates, and special working conditions. An unrestricted area is one that is not under control of the license and is open to the public. The exposure rate must not exceed 2 mrem/h and 100 mrem/y (20μSv/h and 1 mSv/y). Examples are the reception area, the waiting room at the entrance of the NM department, and the hallways around the department. Restricted areas are those under the control of the license. Restricted areas must be posted with radiation warning signs. Figure 3.4 shows two authorized radiation warning signs. A description of warning signs follows.

1. **CAUTION, RADIATION AREA**: An area in which the dose rate could exceed 5 mrem/h (50 μSv/h) at 30 cm from a source.
2. **CAUTION, HIGH-RADIATION AREA**: An area in which the dose rate could exceed 100 mrem/h (1 mSv/h) at 30 cm from any radioactive source. This level is rarely encountered in nuclear medicine.
3. **DANGER, VERY-HIGH-RADIATION AREA**: An area in which the dose rate may reach 500 rem/h (5 Sv/hr) at 1 m from any radioactive source. This case does not apply to nuclear medicine.
4. **CAUTION, RADIOACTIVE MATERIALS**: Any area, room, cabinet, or refrigerator, where significant amounts of radionuclides are stored or used. This sign is required when the minimum activities are as follows:

1 μCi (37 kBq):	^{90}Sr
10 μCi (370 kBq):	^{125}I
100 μCi (3.7 MBq):	^{32}P, ^{90}Y, and ^{137}Cs
1 mCi (37 MBq):	^{57}Co, ^{99}Mo, ^{123}I, ^{131}I, ^{186}Re, and ^{188}Re
10 mCi (370 MBq):	^{11}C, ^{18}F, ^{67}Ga, ^{68}Ga, ^{99m}Tc, and ^{133}Xe

5. **CAUTION, AIRBORNE RADIOACTIVITY**: Placed in any area where radioactive gases, vapors, or dust mixed with the air and averaged over 1 week may exceed 25% of the derived air concentrations (DACs).

PROBLEMS

This set of problems consists of questions on radioactive decay, effect of distance, shielding, and conversion of units. Students may consult Chapter 6 to solve some of these problems.

1. A vial contains a total 65 MBq of ^{123}I solution at 8:00 a.m. How long will it take for the activity to decay to 50 MBq?
2. What percentage of the original radioactivity remains after five half-lives?
3. The count rate of a source at 30 cm from the detector is 480 c/s. At what distance would the count rate reach 660 c/s?
4. While preparing a radiopharmaceutical, a technologist holds a multidose vial with 9-in. forceps for 2 min. The actual distance to the technologist's hand is 7 in. A dosimeter placed on the hand gives a net total dose of 180 μSv after that operation. What would the total dose be if both time and distance were doubled?
5. The dose rate on the surface of a ^{99m}Tc generator is 160 μSv/h. What thickness of additional lead shielding would reduce the dose rate to 20 μSv/h in accordance with ALARA?
6. What percentage of the intensity of a collimated gamma beam would pass through five half-value layers of lead between the source and the detector?
7. For a dosage of 750 MBq, what volume must be drawn from a vial that contains a concentration of 525 MBq/ml?
8. The concentration of an ^{111}In solution is 480 MBq/ml on Monday noon. What would the concentration be at 2:00 p.m. the next day?
9. The concentration of a ^{67}Ga solution is 80 MBq/ml at 8:00 a.m. What volume will contain 50 MBq at 12 noon the same day?
10. The concentration of a ^{131}I solution is 322 MBq/ml on Monday noon. What is the concentration 72 h later?

REFERENCES

Bernier, D.R., Christian, P.E., and Langan, J.K., *Nuclear Medicine Technology and Techniques*, 3d ed., Mosby, St. Louis, 1994.

Bethge, K. et al., *Medical Applications of Nuclear Physics*, Springer–Verlag, Berlin, 2004.

Bevalacqua, J.J., *Basic Health Physics — Problems and Solutions*, Wiley–VCH, Weinheim, 1999.

Chandra, R., *Nuclear Medicine Physics — The Basics*, 6th ed., Lippincott Williams & Wilkins, Philadelphia, 2004.

Code of Federal Regulations, Title 10, National Archives and Records Administration, Washington, DC, 2005.

Dowd, S.B. and Tilson, E.R., *Practical Radiation Protection and Applied Radiobiology*, 2d ed., Saunders, Philadelphia, 1999.

Early, P.J. and Sodee, D.B., *Principles and Practice of Nuclear Medicine*, 2d ed., Mosby, St. Louis, 1995.

Early, P.J., *Review of Rules and Regulations Governing the Practice of Nuclear Medicine*, Orlando, 41st Annual Meeting of the Society of Nuclear Medicine, 1994.

Klingensmith, W.C., Eshima, D., and Goddard, J., *Nuclear Medicine Procedure Manual*, Oxford Medical, Englewood, NJ, 1991.

Kowalsky, R.J. and Falen, S.W., *Radiopharmaceuticals in Nuclear Pharmacy and Nuclear Medicine*, 2d ed., American Pharmacists Association, Washington, DC, 2004.

Mason, J.S., Elliott, K.M., and Mitro, A.C., *The Nuclear Medicine Handbook for Achieving Compliance with NRC Regulations*, Society of Nuclear Medicine, Reston, VA, 1997.

NCRP Report 116, *Limitation of Exposure to Ionizing Radiation*, National Council on Radiation Protection and Measurements, Bethesda, MD, 1993.

Noz, M.E. and Maguire, G.Q., *Radiation Protection in the Radiologic and Health Sciences*, 2d ed., Lea and Febiger, Philadelphia, 1995.

Saha, G.B., *Fundamentals of Nuclear Pharmacy*, 3d ed., Springer–Verlag, New York, 1992.

Saha, G.B., *Physics and Radiobiology of Nuclear Medicine*, Springer–Verlag, New York, 1993.

Saha, G.B., *Basics of PET Imaging*, Springer, New York, 2005.

Sandler, M.P., Coleman, R.E., Patton, J.A., Wackers, F.J., and Gottsckalk, A., Editors, *Diagnostic Nuclear Medicine*, Lippincott Williams & Wilkins, Philadelphia, 2003.

Shleien, B., Slaback, Jr., L.A., and Birky, B.K., Editors, *Handbook of Health Physics and Radiological Health*, 3d ed., Lippincott Williams & Wilkins, Philadelphia, 1998.

Slater, R.J., *Radioisotopes in Biology*, 2d ed., Oxford University Press, Englewood, NJ, 2002.

Statkiewics-Sherer, M.A., Visconti, P.J., and Ritenour, E.R., *Radiation Protection in Medical Radiography*, 2d ed., Mosby, St. Louis, 1993.

Steves, A.M., *Review of Nuclear Medicine Technology*, 2d ed., Society of Nuclear Medicine, Reston, VA, 1996.

Turner, J.E., Editor, *Atoms, Radiation, and Radiation Protection*, 2d ed., John Wiley and Sons, New York, 1995.

4 Radiation Detection and Measurement

I. RATIONALE

To plan and to practice radiation safety, NMTs and NMT students must familiarize themselves with three kinds of instrumentation: (a) nonimaging instruments: well-type scintillation counters, thyroid uptake systems, and dose calibrators, (b) imaging instrumentation: gamma cameras, SPECT cameras, and PET/CT scanners, and (c) survey instruments to monitor and maintain a safe radiation level in the NM department: GM (Geiger–Muller) survey meters, room alarm monitors, and personal alarm monitors; and ionization chambers (cutie pies, dose calibrators, pocket dosimeters). In this chapter, the basic principles of design and operation of those instruments are discussed briefly. For a more profound study of the engineering and operation of NM equipment, readers are referred to the specialized literature.

To maintain a safe working environment in the NM department, NMTs must operate the monitoring instruments correctly, maintain them in proper order by performing timely quality assurance (QA) testings, and monitor the department as mandated by the NRC or the licensing agency. Furthermore, records of QA tests and monitoring results must be kept and made available during inspections by a licensing agency representative. For surveys and monitoring techniques, see also Chapter 7.

II. FUNDAMENTALS

A. Principles

Ionizing radiations cannot be seen, heard, smelled, tasted, or touched. Alpha, beta, gamma, x-rays, and neutrons (n) are radiations that cannot be perceived by human senses. Consequently, indirect approaches must be used to detect or measure those radiations. The best and most practical approach is one in which the energy of those radiations is converted into an electrical signal. That electrical signal can be in the form of a "pulse" or in the form of a continuous current. A single detected event can be registered as a *count*, and the number of counts registered per unit time is the *count rate*, such as counts per minute (c/min) or counts per second (c/s). The basic scheme is

$$\text{Energy} \longrightarrow \text{Detector} \longrightarrow \text{Electrical signal}$$

$$(\alpha, \beta, \gamma, \text{X}, \text{n}) \quad \text{(Gas, liquid, solid)} \quad \text{(Pulse, count, current)}$$

B. Detection

Detection of radiation is a qualitative observation that may result in the presence or absence of radiation above the normal background. Detection does not require accuracy. Results are either positive or negative to the presence of radioactivity.

C. Radioactive Contamination

In general, contamination is the unintentional spill or release of radioactivity in some area of the NM department. Low-level contamination involves quantities of a few nanocuries (a few hundred becquerels) to a few microcuries (a few hundred kilobecquerels) of radioactivity. High-level contamination means the release of a millicurie (37 MBq) or more. Careful workers maintain their imaging rooms, imaging instrumentation, lab counters, fume hoods, etc., free from contamination; that is, surveys result in radiation levels that are indistinguishable from background radiation levels.

D. Measurement

Measurement is a quantitative observation. In this case, accuracy is required. For example, when preparing a dosage of a radiopharmaceutical for a patient, extreme care must be exercised to ensure an accurate dosage.

E. Radiation Survey Instruments

Some instruments are designed for detection only. Other instruments are designed for measurements. A brief introduction follows. See also Chapter 7.

1. Gas Detectors

a. Geiger–Muller (GM) portable survey meters: Used in laboratory surveys (detection).
b. Portable ionization chambers: Portable survey instruments used in low- to high-level exposure rate monitorings, especially in radiopharmacies.
c. Pocket dosimeters: Small ionization chambers used in personnel exposure monitoring. Some of these are GM counters and may have an alarm setting.
d. Wipe-test counters: GM counters specially designed to decide whether or not a wipe comes from a contaminated area.
e. Area alarm monitors: GM counters designed to sound an alarm at some set count rate.
f. Dose calibrators: Large well-type ionization chambers used mostly to assay elution products from generators and to prepare diagnostic and therapeutic dosages of radiopharmaceuticals for patients. Specially

designed dose calibrators are used for PET RPs. Others are specially designed for beta emitters used in radionuclide therapy.

2. Personal Exposure Monitors

X-ray film badges, thermoluminescent dosimeter (TLD) badges, and TLD ring dosimeters are used to measure personnel whole-body and extremity radiation doses.

3. Scintillation Detectors

a. Portable scintillation survey detectors: Solid detectors, usually made of Na(Tl) crystals. They are used in radiation surveys of laboratory surfaces and in wipe monitoring.
b. Well-type single-channel analyzers (SCAs): Used in measurement of laboratory and instrument wipes and swabs from leak-testing of sealed sources. Extremely sensitive and accurate, they are also used in nonimaging procedures.
c. Multichannel gamma ray spectrometers, also known as multichannel analyzers (MCAs): Used in the identification and quantification of gamma contaminants.

F. Interpretation

Surveying or monitoring for radioactive contamination means comparing observations with the normal levels of background. Because both vary in a random fashion, low-level contaminations may require statistical methods for proper interpretation. Instruction on basic statistics is included later in this chapter.

III. GAS DETECTORS

A. Basic Design

1. Components

Gas detectors consist of a gas-filled (air, CO_2, or argon), cylinder-shaped chamber containing two electrodes (anode and cathode), connected to a power supply (battery), which provides the needed voltage for operation. The circuit may include a series of resistors to expand the scale of readings and an electrometer to read the current. The readout may be analog or digital. The scales may be calibrated to give readings in c/min, mR/h, or μSv/h. Figure 4.1 shows the basic design of a gas detector.

2. Ions Collected and Voltage

In general, the number of ions collected in all gas detectors varies with the applied voltage. GM counters collect ions in the form of pulses or counts; ion chambers collect ions in the form of a continuous current. Figure 4.2 shows the typical

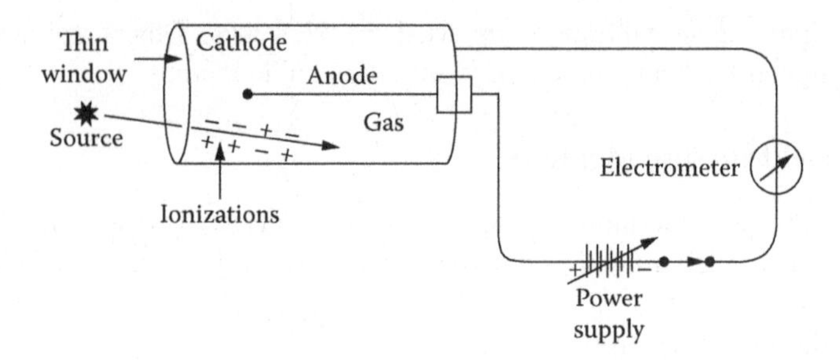

FIGURE 4.1 Diagram of cylindrical gas detector and its associated electrical circuit. This basic design is similar in all gas detectors.

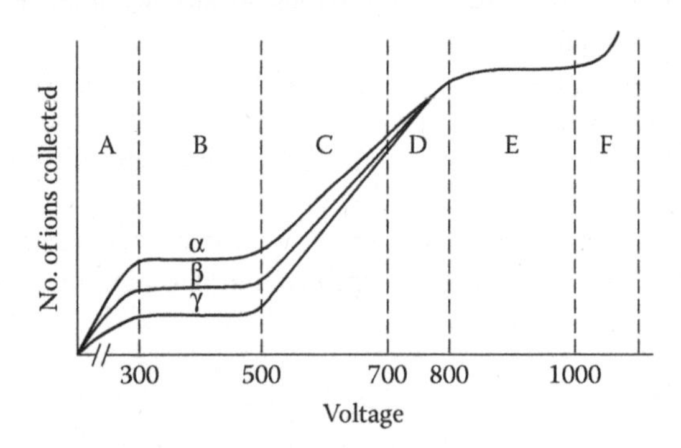

FIGURE 4.2 Gas detector responses for alpha, beta, and gamma radiations as a function of applied voltage. The most important regions are B, the ionization chamber region; C, the proportional region; and E, the Geiger–Muller region.

responses of gas detectors. In the figure, various regions are recognized. Voltages are approximate:

a. Region A: recombination region. The applied voltage is not high enough for collection of ions at the electrodes. They readily recombine.
b. Region B: ionization chamber region. The voltage is high enough to separate and collect ions at the corresponding electrodes. Only primary ions are produced and collected. Pocket dosimeters, cutie pies, and dose calibrators operate in this region.
c. Region C: proportionality region. The applied voltage is strong enough to produce acceleration of ions that interact with gas atoms or molecules, causing secondary ionizations. This effect increases linearly with the applied voltage. Proportional counters operate in this region. They are used by environmentalists to measure very low levels of alpha emitters such as plutonium-239 and radium-226 in water and beta emitters such as ^{131}I, ^{90}Sr, ^{14}C, and ^{3}H in air and water samples.
d. Region D: limited proportionality region. This is only a transition region.
e. Region E: GM region. This region shows a plateau; the number of ions collected is fairly constant despite the voltage increase in the region. Every

detection event results in an avalanche of ions regardless of the energy of the radiation that started it. The slope of the plateau is an index of the quality of the GM tube. High quality means a slope of less than 10% per 100 V. It takes between 200 and 300 μs for a GM detector to recover from each event. That time is known as the *resolving time*. On the high side of the plateau, continuous discharge is possible. To prevent continuous discharges, a quenching gas can be added to the argon in the tube. Organic quenched tubes might contain ethanol vapor, and inorganic quenched tubes could contain chlorine gas. GM beta–gamma survey meters operate in this region. Some GM detectors may be equipped with a sound alarm system which can be set at 10 or 20 mR/h (100 or 200 μSv/h). They are very useful in hot labs and commercial radiopharmacies.

f. Region F: continuous discharge region. The applied voltage is too high for operation.

B. GM Survey Meters

1. Design

GM survey meters are specially designed for laboratory surveying. They can detect microcurie (kBq) levels of beta and gamma emitters provided that their energies vary from medium to high. Most NM radionuclides fall in this category. For nanocurie (becquerel) levels or low energies, the wipe-technique is recommended, as long as measurements are done with liquid scintillation counters for beta emitters and well-type NaI(Tl) crystal counters for gamma emitters.

2. Scales

GM counters have adjustable scales to read 0 to 2 mR/h, 0 to 20 mR/h, 0 to 200 mR/h, and some may even have 0 to 2 R/h capability. Respectively, those ranges correspond to 0–20 μSv/h, 0–200 μSv/h, 0–2 mSv/h, and 0–20 mSv/h.

3. Wall Thickness

The GM tube wall can be made of glass with a density-thickness of 30 mg/cm^2, excellent for gamma emitters. Those tubes are lined with a bismuth metal compound to increase the detection efficiency for gamma emitters. Some end-window tubes might have a thin mica window of only 4-mg/cm^2 thickness, good for beta emitters.

4. Gases

The gas in the tube can be argon with either 10% ethanol vapor or 1% chlorine for quenching purposes. The life of an organic tube is about 1 billion counts. Inorganic tubes have limitless lives because the chlorine ions recombine.

5. Error of Detection

A GM survey meter calibrated with a ^{137}Cs standard could have an error of plus or minus 10% when surveying for ^{137}Cs. The error may be as high as 20% when surveying for other radionuclides. That is acceptable because they are detecting instruments, not measuring instruments.

6. Time Constant

The electrical circuit of GM survey meters comes with a variable resistor that allows the user to change the time constant (TC) of the instrument. Short TCs are used for a fast response. Long TCs are used when a slow response is sufficient.

7. Disadvantage

At very high levels of radiation, the GM counter may "go blank." This cannot happen in an NM department because the levels are never that high.

C. Calibration of GM Survey Meters

1. Sealed Source

Some survey meters come with a small radium-226 sealed source, which can be used to check the instrument for proper response at some fixed distance. Read the manual. If the response is correct, the monitoring of the laboratory can proceed.

2. Regulation

As per NRC or state regulations (10CFR20.1501), survey meters must be recalibrated annually by a certified instrumentation expert.

3. Correction Factor

Calibration means to adjust the response of the instrument to the expected exposure rate at some fixed distance from a certified standard source. Sources used in this procedure are usually ^{226}Ra or ^{137}Cs. The expected exposure rate is calculated using the specific gamma constant. See Table 2.3. An alternate approach is to generate a correction factor (CF), derived as follows:

$$CF = \frac{\text{Expected count rate}}{\text{Observed count rate}}$$

a. Calibration is usually done for all scales, at the low and high sides of each scale, and for up to 1000 mR/h (10 mSv/h).
b. A certificate of calibration is issued by the person who performs the calibration. A sticker showing the CF may be placed on the side of the instrument.
c. The user must multiply observed readings by the CF before entering results in the radiation survey records.

D. Wipe-Test Counters

1. Design

These are instruments designed to measure the activity in "wipes" obtained from laboratory surfaces: tables, counters, fume hoods, stretchers, imaging tables, gamma cameras, floors, etc. They are also used to measure swabs from leak-tests of sealed sources. Each wipe usually covers about 100 cm^2 of wiped area (a circle of about 11.3 cm in diameter).

2. Positive Wipes

Wipe-test counters are actually thin end-window GM counters that can be calibrated with a small ^{137}Cs source. Any wipe exceeding a preset count rate contains more than 2200 disintegrations per minute (DPM) per 100 cm^2 and is, therefore, considered positive.

E. Portable Ionization Chambers

1. Properties

Better known as cutie pies, these are high-level, slow-response radiation survey instruments and are best suited for hot labs and radiopharmacies, where curie-level generators (GBq-level) may be used. The gas in the chamber may be dry air or CO_2.

2. Accuracy

Readouts can be analog or digital. Because they operate at low voltages, only primary ions are collected, which makes them very precise and accurate instruments.

3. Scales

Typical readout scales cover a wide range of readings, from 0–5 mR/h (0–50 μSv/h) to 0–50 R/h (0–500 mSv/h). A similar procedure to that given above for GM counters can be used to verify the proper operation of ion chambers. In practice, a battery check and an adjustment of the zero reading is sufficient to start monitoring.

F. Dose Calibrators

1. Accurate Assays

Dose calibrators are the "workhorses" of the NM department. They are well-type ionization chambers, extremely useful in the assay of generator eluants, ^{99}Mo breakthrough measurements, preparation of radiopharmaceuticals, and dispensing dosages of RPs for patients. Some dose calibrators are specially designed for beta emitters, and some for PET RPs.

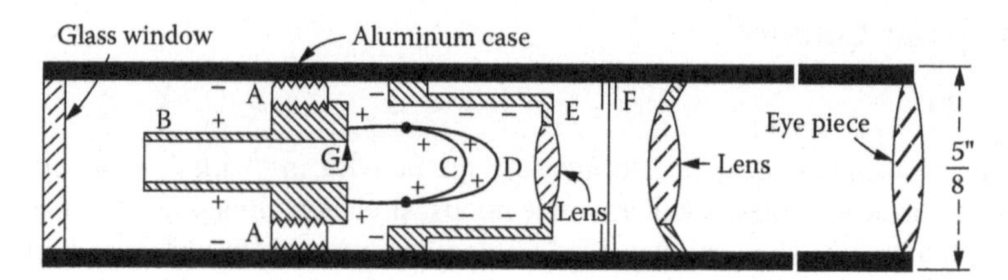

FIGURE 4.3 Pocket dosimeter. Components: A, insulating ring; B, charging rod; C, fixed metal-coated quartz fiber; D, movable metal-coated quartz fiber; E, metal cylinder; F, transparent scale; and G, metal support.

2. Safety

Indirectly, dose calibrators ensure the safety of radiopharmacists and NM technologists because they are quick and accurate, thus reducing the time of exposure.

G. Pocket Dosimeters

1. Design

Some pocket dosimeters are ionization chambers that are the shape and size of a pen; they are used to measure the total radiation dose received by radiation workers during some time interval. They cover the range of 0–500 mrem (0–5 mSv). Other pocket dosimeters are actually GM counters with a range of 0–50 mrem/h (0–500 μSv/h).

2. Operation

The dosimeter operates like a condenser. An electrical charge is applied to load the condenser. Gamma or x-rays cause discharge of the condenser. The dose received is read on a calibrated scale. Figure 4.3 shows the components of a pocket dosimeter. The applied charge separates the two metal-coated quartz fibers by electrical repulsion, just as in an electroscope. Discharge of the fibers makes one of them move across the scale.

3. Applications

Depending on need, the user might wear the dosimeter in the chest pocket for a whole-body dose measurement, on the wrist for a hand dose, or inside a lead apron for a fetal dose in case of a declared pregnancy.

4. Advantage

An advantage of these dosimeters is their immediate reading. A dosimeter may be taped to the dorsal part of the hand, or placed inside the glove, and used during the assay of a generator eluant, preparation of a multidose radiopharmaceutical kit, drawing of a patient dose into hypodermic syringes, or injection of a substance. Having an immediate reading allows technologists to plan their work better toward

TABLE 4.1
Properties of Gas Detectors

Type	Operating Voltage (V)	Ions Collected	Continuous Discharge	Radiations
Ion chambers	50–300	Primary only	No	α, β, γ, X
Proportional counters	500–800	Proportional to voltage	No	α, β
GM counters	800–900	Full avalanche	Yes[a]	β, γ, X

[a] See text for quenching of discharge.

TABLE 4.2
Uses of Gas Detectors

Type	Examples	Uses	Scales	Disadvantages
Ionization chambers	Survey ion chambers	Hot labs	0–50 R/h (0–500 mSv/h)	Slow response
	Pocket dosimeters	Personal monitoring	0–500 mrem (0–5 mSv)	Fragile
	Dose calibrators	Hot labs	1 μCi–10 Ci (37 kBq–70 GBq)	Geometry-dependent
Proportional counters	Gas flow, 4π geometry[a]	Ecological, nuclear reactors	pCi-level, Neutron flux	Requires special training
GM counters	β–γ survey meters	Laboratory monitoring	0–1000 mR/h (0–10 mSv/h)	10–20% error
	GM pocket dosimeters	Personal monitoring	0–50 mR/h(0–500 μSv/h)	None

[a] 4π geometry: The sample is placed inside, at the center, of a spherically shaped detector.

reducing exposures. A disadvantage is that these dosimeters are fragile. Dropping them accidentally can cause loss of the reading.

H. Summary of Gas Detectors

Table 4.1 and Table 4.2 summarize the properties and uses of gas detectors.

IV. SCINTILLATION DETECTORS

A. Basic Design

1. The Na(Tl) Detector

A sodium iodide crystal, activated with thallium, NaI(Tl), coupled to a photomultiplier tube (PMT), is a most efficient gamma detector. Figure 4.4 shows a diagram of a scintillation detector. The iodine in the crystal (atomic number = 53) has a high

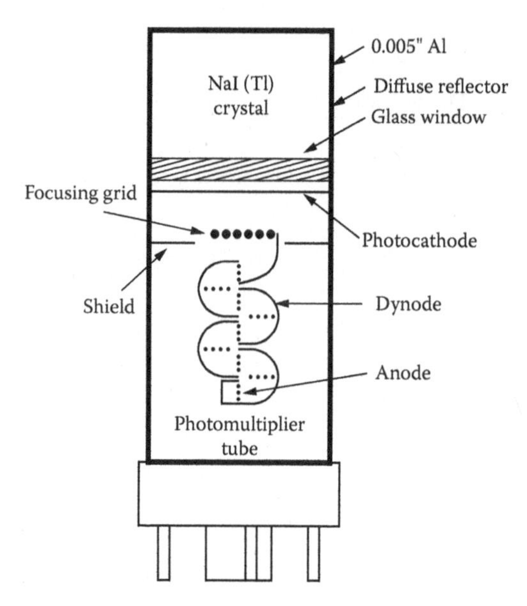

FIGURE 4.4 Gamma scintillation detector: A sodium iodide crystal activated with thallium, NaI(Tl). The crystal is coupled to a photomultiplier tube (PMT).

cross section for gamma ray interactions. The crystal density is 3.67 g/cm^3. Because the crystal is hygroscopic, it must be sealed in an airtight aluminum case.

2. Principle

a. A gamma ray enters the crystal and causes ionization of many iodine atoms. The ejected electrons travel in the conduction band of the crystal. Soon, however, they fall back to the valence band with the emission of ultraviolet photons. Adding thallium to the crystal makes the returning electrons fall in a two-step jump, emitting 4,100-Å photons (blue-violet) perfectly compatible with the PMT.
b. The blue-violet photons enter the PMT through a glass window and hit the cathode, which is made of a Cs_3Sb compound, where they release many electrons by photoelectric effect. The number of electrons is then multiplied by jumping through 10 to 12 dynodes having increasing voltages applied to them. The dynodes are coated with Cs_3Sb. Depending on the voltage applied to the PMT, the signal reaching the anode could have an amplitude of 100 mV. The signal will then be amplified for processing and counting.

B. Associated Electronics

1. Single-Channel Analyzer (SCA)

Figure 4.5 shows the components of a single-channel gamma ray spectrometer, which processes and counts signals. The output signal from the PMT enters the

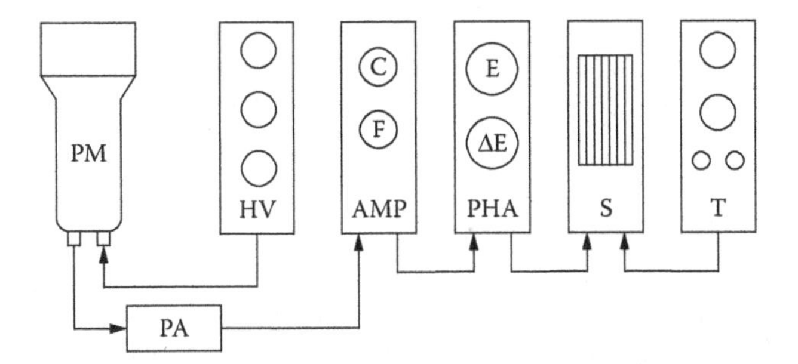

FIGURE 4.5 Gamma ray spectrometer. Modular components: the detector (left); PA: preamplifier; HV: high-voltage power supply; AMP: amplifier; C: coarse gain; F: fine gain; PHA: pulse height analyzer; S: scaler; T: timer.

preamplifier, which acts as an efficient coupler between the PMT and the main amplifier. The main amplifier is used to increase the pulse height to a suitable amplitude during calibration.

2. The Window

Applying two electronic discriminators, the analyzer selects a narrow band of signal amplitudes for counting. The scaler is an electronic counter, and the timer is an electronic clock.

3. Applications

a. Single-channel analyzers (SCA) and multichannel analyzers (MCA) can be used to measure samples from blood volume determinations, Schilling tests, red blood cell survival tests, as well as wipes from laboratory monitoring and swabs from leak-testing of sealed sources.
b. Portable scintillation area survey instruments are very sensitive at detecting gamma-emitting radionuclides in the hot lab, imaging rooms, patient beds, etc.

4. Other Scintillation Detectors

Some imaging systems (SPECT) use BGO (bismuth germanate) crystals, and PET scanners may use either BGO or LSO (lithium oxyorthosilicate) crystals, which have a better stopping power for annihilation radiation photons. A brief description of NM imaging systems follows.

V. IMAGING INSTRUMENTATION

Noninvasive NM imaging procedures have provided physicians with functional images of organ systems for several decades. The advances made in recent years, particularly in positron emission tomography (PET), have been remarkable. Some of the NM imaging systems are briefly described here.

A. Conventional Imaging

1. Planar Imaging

Patients referred to NM may be subjected to a planar imaging study, which involves the recording of multiple views of the distribution of the radioactivity within the body at some time after injection. The images are a two-dimensional (2D) representation of what is really a three-dimensional (3D) distribution and, therefore, imperfect. This is because of the overlaying of sources within the body and the attenuation of photons within the same.

2. SPECT

Some patients may be sent for a SPECT study (single-photon emission computerized tomography), which depicts coronal, sagittal, and transversal sections of the body to provide a 3D representation. The computer can then produce time–activity curves of selected regions of interest (ROIs) from any slice or from multiple slices on record. "Gated SPECT" depicts movie loops of blood as it passes through the chambers of the heart. "Dynamic SPECT" shows chemical changes in organs or tissues as a function of time.

B. Pet Imaging

1. Metabolic Tracers

PET radiopharmaceuticals (RPs) truly represent the definition of biological tracers. They depict function without pharmacological action on the patient. And their concentration in tissues is proportional to metabolic rate. Because they trace molecules, they also fall within the domain of the emerging field of molecular medicine. Table 4.3 shows the main properties of some PET radionuclides of interest in NM. Table 4.4 gives the indications of some PET imaging RPs.

TABLE 4.3
PET Radionuclides

Radionuclide	Half-Life	E_{max} (keV)	Production
^{18}F	110 min	635	Cyclotron
^{68}Ga	68 min	1880	$^{68}Ge/^{68}Ga$ generator
^{11}C	20 min	970	Cyclotron
^{13}N	10 min	1190	Cyclotron
^{15}O	2 min	1700	Cyclotron
^{82}Rb	75 sec	3350	$^{82}Sr/^{82}Rb$ generator

TABLE 4.4
Radiopharmaceuticals for PET

	Indications
^{18}F-FDG	Imaging of coronary artery disease and left ventricular dysfunction, imaging of head, neck, esophageal, breast, and colorectal cancers and melanomas, study of epileptic seizures
^{13}N-ammonia	Myocardial perfusion at rest and exercise
^{82}Rb-chloride	Myocardial perfusion
^{11}C-acetate	Regional myocardial blood flow, reflects oxidative metabolism; prostatic cancer imaging
^{18}F-fluorodopa	Imaging of brain dopamine neurons, imaging of patients with Parkinson's and Huntington's diseases
^{15}O-water	Myocardial blood flow studies

2. The PET Scanner

a. A PET scanner consists of multiple rings of bismuth germanate (BGO) or lutetium oxyorthosilicate (LSO) crystal detectors arranged around the patient. The patient receives an intravenous injection of the prescribed PET imaging agent. The 511 keV photons emitted upon positron annihilation within the patient's body are detected by crystal detectors 180 degrees apart wired in electronic coincidence. This process is also known as "electronic collimation."
b. The rings of detectors move along the length of the patient's body during acquisition. The computer makes corrections for attenuation, random events, dead-time, scatter, etc. as part of the reconstruction process, and then it displays sectional and/or 3D images.
c. The interpretation of the images requires reference to a metabolic model.

C. The Merging of PET and CT

1. Computerized Tomography (CT)

CT is a radiological procedure in which an x-ray tube encircles the patient, emitting x-rays through the body. A ring of crystal detectors measures the transmitted intensities, and a computer calculates the attenuation coefficients. Applying a grayscale, it reconstructs a sectional image. Helical rotation of the x-ray tube allows acquisition of data for a portion of the body or the whole body. The computer reconstructs sectional or 3D images. The images show exquisite anatomical resolution.

2. Coverage

In recent years, the expansion of Medicare coverage for PET imaging procedures has resulted in a multiplication of PET centers in the United States. These centers have medical cyclotrons to produce the radionuclides needed and radiochemical synthesizers to prepare the imaging agents. PET centers can then supply hospitals, within a metropolitan area, the necessary RPs for PET imaging.

3. The PET/CT Scanner

This device consists of a PET scanner and a CT scanner assembled in tandem. Such device or hybrid scanner, as it is sometimes called, may have a 16-slice capability and may scan the whole body in less than 8 min. Needless to say, that is of utmost importance to the patient. The PET and the CT images can be displayed side by side or superimposed on each other (alignment) for interpretation.

4. Applications

PET/CT imaging procedures help physicians differentiate ischemic from infarcted myocardium, benign from malignant tumors, stage cancers, monitor the response to therapy, and diagnose Alzheimer's in the early stages of the disease, among others. Furthermore, high resolution PET/CT scanners (2 mm) are being used in the evaluation of new PET RPs for efficacy and safety in laboratory animals.

VI. STATISTICS OF COUNTING

Radioactive atoms decay at random, independently from each other. For that reason, all measurements of radioactivity have an inherent, uncontrollable random error.

A. Types of Errors

1. Systematic Errors

Systematic errors are due to a defect in the method of observation. They are controllable by the repair or replacement of the method.

2. Random Errors

Random errors are variations inherent to the phenomenon being observed. They are uncontrollable. An example is radioactive decay.

3. Blunders

These are errors due to carelessness, negligence, or ignorance, and are controllable.

B. Statistical Distributions

1. Poisson Distribution

This is a bell-shaped curve that best describes the frequencies of radioactivity measurements around the mean value. The curve is slightly asymmetric and skewed toward the high values.

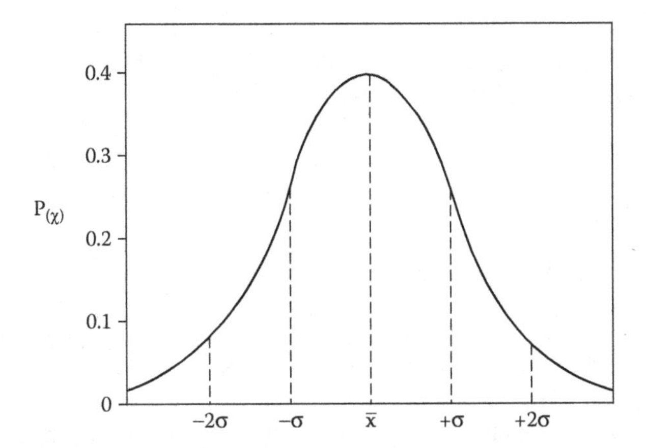

FIGURE 4.6 Normal (Gaussian) distribution. The curve is symmetrical and its parameters are $\overline{x}$, the mean, and σ, the standard deviation. $P_{(X)}$ is the probability of individual observations.

2. Gaussian Distribution

The Gaussian distribution, also known as *normal distribution*, is a close approximation to the Poisson distribution. The curve is symmetrical and, for that reason, easier to use. Its parameters are m, the true mean, and s, the standard deviation.

C. The Normal Distribution

1. Sample

Sample is a limited number of observations. In a sample, the arithmetic mean, $\overline{x}$, is a close approximation to the true mean (Figure 4.6). The sample mean and the sample standard deviation, σ_s, can be calculated as follows:

$$\overline{x} = \Sigma x_i / n \tag{4.1}$$

$$\sigma_s = [\Sigma(X_i - \overline{x})^2 / (n-1)]^{1/2} \tag{4.2}$$

where σ_s = sample standard deviation, Σ = sum of, X_i = each individual observation, and n = number of observations in the sample.

2. Ranges of Confidence

a. In a sample, 68.3% of the observations fall within the mean ± σ_s. This is the 68% confidence range. The odds that a new observation will fall in that range are 2/3 in favor and 1/3 against.

b. In a sample, 95.5% of the observations fall within the mean ± $2\sigma_s$. This is the 95% confidence range. The odds that a new observation will fall in that range are 21/22 in favor and 1/22 against.
c. In a sample, 99.7% of the observations fall within the mean ± $3\sigma_s$. This is the 99% confidence range. The odds that a new observation will fall within that range are 332/333 in favor and 1/333 against.

3. The Meaning of σ_s

a. The sample standard deviation is an expression of the random error in a series of replicate counts of a long-lived radioactive source. It is also an expression of the spread of the data around the mean.
b. The sample standard deviation allows the prediction of where a single new observation would fall in the normal distribution.

4. Practical Rules

a. The standard deviation of a single observation is the square root of the total counts. For example, if 40,000 counts are collected in 10 min, then we can report the result as 40,000 ± 200 c/10 min; 200 is the square root of 40,000.
b. The standard deviation of a count rate (σ_R) is the square root of the total counts divided by the counting time. In the previous example, the count rate and its standard deviation are 4,000 ± 20 c/min.

5. Background Radiation

a. When background (Bkg) count rate is less than 1% of the source gross count rate, it may be ignored. Most NM observations fall in this category.
b. When Bkg count rate is greater than 1% but less than 10% of the source gross count rate, it must be subtracted to obtain the net count rate. In NM, many observations fall into this category.
c. If Bkg count rate is greater than 10% of the source gross count rate, the standard deviation of the net count rate (σ_R) can be calculated using the following formula:

$$\sigma_R = [(R_g/t_g) + (R_b/t_b)]^{1/2} \tag{4.3}$$

where R_g = gross count rate of the source, t_g = counting time of the source, R_b = background count rate, and t_b = counting time of background.

Sample Problem

A Schilling test urine sample results in a count of 1600 c/10 min. Bkg count is 1,800 c/20 min. What is the net count rate and its standard deviation?

Solution: First, sample gross count rate: 1600/10 = 160 c/min. Second, Bkg count rate: 1800/20 = 90 c/min. Third, net sample count rate: 160 – 90 = 70 c/min. Fourth, for σ_R, use Equation 4.3. Result: ±4.53 c/min. Report: 70 ± 5 c/min (answer).

6. Coefficient of Variation (CV)

The coefficient of variation is the sample standard deviation expressed as a percentage of the mean. The CV is a measure of precision or reproducibility:

$$CV = \sigma_s \times 100 / \bar{x}$$

7. Standard Deviation of the Mean, $\sigma_{\bar{x}}$

Also called *standard error*, the standard deviation of the mean allows the prediction of the new mean if the whole series of observations were to be repeated. The formula is

$$\sigma_{\bar{x}} = [(\Sigma(X_i - \bar{x})^2 / n(n-1)]^{1/2} \quad (4.4)$$

8. Total Counts Collected (N)

Collecting the highest total counts within a reasonable time increases the reliability of any observation. Table 4.5 shows the decrease in the CV with an increase in the total counts collected.

9. Reliability

Most medical studies are aimed at the 95% confidence range. Most radioactivity measurements are aimed at a CV of 1%.

Sample Problem

How many counts (N) must be collected for a ± 2% error at the 95% confidence level?

Solution: Formula for the 95% confidence: N = 40,000/% error^2. Substituting: N = 40,000/2^2 = 10,000 counts (answer).

Note: If 2% represents 2σ, then σ = 1%; Table 4.5 gives also 10,000 counts.

TABLE 4.5
Reducing the Statistical Error

Total Counts	Standard Deviation	CV (%)
100	10	10
1000	31.6	3.16
5000	70.7	1.4
10000	100	1.0
25000	158.1	0.63
40000	200	0.5

10. Rejection of Data

In a set of observations (sample), one or more observations can be rejected if they fall outside of the 95% confidence range (outside of the mean $\pm 2\sigma$). The *Chauvenet's criterion* for rejection of data contends that the rejection level is a function of the number of observations, n, and gives the following limits:

n	Limit, σ_s
5	1.64
10	1.97
20	2.24
100	2.80

Sample Problem

In the following sample, can any of the observations be rejected: 530, 490, 510, 480, and 520 c/min? The mean and the sample standard deviation are 506 ± 21.
Solution: The limits are set at $1.64 \times 21 = 34$ or $506 \pm 34 = 472$ to 540. None can be rejected (answer).

VII. MAKING DECISIONS

A. Relative Error (τ)

1. Detector Performance

Repetitive countings of a long-lived source, made with a detector, should not vary more than the expected random decay of the source. If they do, the detector is at fault. The relative error is a way to decide if the detector is working properly.

Sample Problem

A long-lived source is counted twice with a GM counter. Results are 10,690 c/10 min and 10,100 c/10 min. Is the counter operating properly?
Solution: Apply the relative error formula:

$$\tau = (R_1 - R_2)/[(R_1/t_1) + (R_2/t_2)]^{1/2} \tag{4.5}$$

where R_1, R_2 = the two count rates and t_1, t_2 = the two counting times.

The relative error (τ) is expressed in the number of standard deviations. No more than 2.5 standard deviations are accepted (1% probability) as a random variation.

Substituting the two count rates and the two counting times in Equation 4.5 results in a relative error of 4.09 standard deviations. This value is taken to Table 4.6 to show that 4.09 falls outside the table and has a probability of less than 1% of being due to the random decay of the source only. Therefore, it is unlikely that the difference is just a random variation. Conclusion: The difference is due to improper operation of the counter (answer).

TABLE 4.6
Probabilities (*P*) of Relative Errors

Relative Error (Number of SDs)[a]	*P* (%)	Relative Error (Number of SDs)[a]	*P* (%)
0.0	100.0	1.4	16.2
0.1	92.0	1.5	13.4
0.2	84.1	1.6	11.0
0.3	76.4	1.7	9.0
0.4	68.9	1.8	7.2
0.5	61.7	1.9	6.0
0.6	54.8	2.0	4.6
0.7	48.3	2.1	3.6
0.8	42.3	2.2	2.8
0.9	36.8	2.3	2.2
1.0	31.7	2.4	1.6
1.1	27.2	2.5	1.24
1.2	23.0	2.6	0.93
1.3	19.4		

[a] SD = Standard deviation.

2. Is There Contamination?

To decide whether or not there is contamination, surveys, wipes, and swabs count rates must be compared with background count rates. The use of the relative error is useful.

Sample Problems

a. A wipe obtained from the face of a gamma camera results in 455 counts/10 min.
   Background count rate is 400 c/10 min. Is the camera contaminated?
   Solution: Applying the relative error formula results in 1.88 standard deviations. Table 4.6 gives a probability of 6%, a very likely random difference. No, the camera is not contaminated (answer).
b. In the radioassay laboratory, a piece of glassware yields 48 c/2 min. Bkg is 240 c/20 min. Is the glassware contaminated?
   Solution: In this case, the relative error is 3.38 standard deviations. Table 4.6 gives a probability of less than 1% to this result. That is unacceptable. Therefore, the glassware is contaminated.

VIII. MINIMUM DETECTABLE ACTIVITY (MDA)

MDA is the smallest amount of radioactivity that can be measured reliably with a counter at the 99% confidence level. To determine the MDA of a counter, a standard (NBS, or NBS-traceable) is needed.

Sample Problem

Determine the MDA of a well-type gamma counter. A 0.1-μCi ^{137}Cs NBS standard yields a net count rate of 7500 c/min. A 20-min background count results in 1,200 c/20 min or 60 c/min.

Solution: The MDA is calculated as follows:

$$\text{MDA} = \frac{3(\text{Bkg}/\text{t})^{1/2}}{\text{c}/\text{min}\ \mu\text{Ci}} \tag{4.6}$$

where Bkg = count rate of Bkg or 60 c/min; t = counting time of Bkg or 20 min; and c/min/μCi = counts per minute per microcurie of the standard. Substituting

$$[3(60/20)^{1/2}]/(7{,}500/0.1) = 6.9 \times 10^{-5}\ \mu\text{Ci (answer)}.$$

Note: Well-type gamma counters are remarkable instruments. In the example, the instrument can detect 69 picocuries of radioactivity and still distinguish it from background at the 99% level of confidence.

IX. QUALITY ASSURANCE OF RADIATION COUNTERS

A. Reliability

As stated earlier, in a series of replicate counts of a long-lived source, a counter should not vary more than the expected random variations of radioactive decay. If the instrument varies more than the set limits, then it is not operating properly and may have to be repaired or replaced.

B. QA Tests

Very briefly, we can mention the three most important QA tests for reproducibility performed routinely to test the quality of a radiation counter.

1. The Relative Error (τ)

The relative error test is used when only two observations are available. This test was described in Section VII of this chapter (Equation 4.5).

2. The Reliability Factor (RF)

The RF is used when more than two observations are available and is equal to the ratio of the sample standard deviation to the theoretical standard deviation, which, in turn, is equal to the square root of the mean. The RF is a function of the number of observations. Figure 4.7 shows two sets of curves, which represent the limits at two levels of confidence. For example, for ten observations, using the outside set of curves (96% confidence level), the RF acceptable limits are from 0.5 to 1.4.

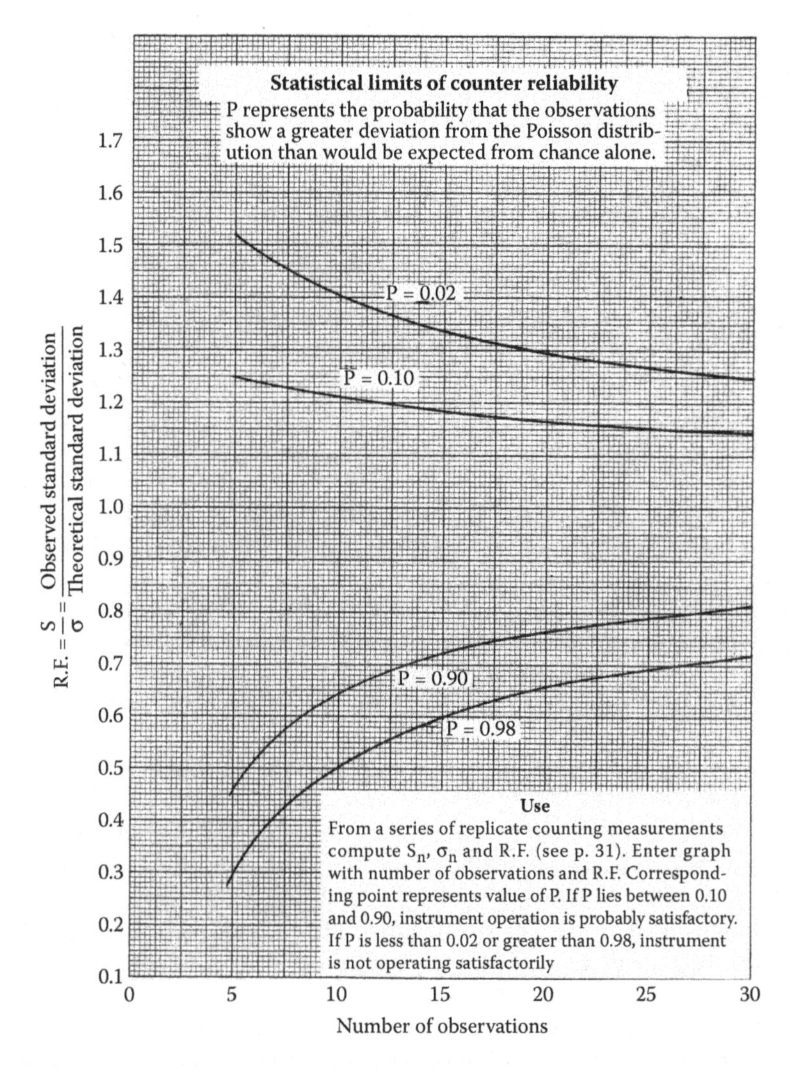

FIGURE 4.7 Instrument reliability factor. A method for assessing the performance of radiation detectors.

3. The Chi-Squared Test (χ^2)

This test is used with 10, 20, or more observations. In NM, 20 observations are routinely used. The chi-squared value is calculated as the sum of all the differences from the mean squared and divided by the mean:

$$\chi^2 = \Sigma(X_i - \overline{x})^2 / \overline{x} \tag{4.7}$$

The calculated chi-squared value is taken to a probability table to decide whether or not it is acceptable. Usually, the value has to fall outside of the 98% confidence range to be considered unacceptable. The limits for n = 5, 10, 20, and 30 are given in the following text:

n	Limits, 98%
5	0.297–13.277
10	2.088–21.666
20	7.633–36.191
30	14.256–49.588

PROBLEMS

1. The gross count rate of a source is 3350 c/5 min. Background is 780 c/10 min. What are the net count rate and its standard deviation?

For Problems 2, 3, 4, and 5, consider the following situation: A series of measurements of a long-lived source resulted in the following observations: 2,654, 2,633, 2,672, 2,598, and 2,648 c/min.

2. Find the arithmetic mean and the sample standard deviation.
3. What is the coefficient of variation and the standard error?
4. Calculate the reliability factor and the chi-squared value. Based on your results, is the radiation counter working properly?
5. Applying the Chauvenet criterion, could any of the observations be rejected?
6. A wipe obtained from the probe of a gamma camera resulted in 986 c/10 min. Background was 1688 c/20 minutes. Is the camera contaminated?
7. The levels of thyroxine in the blood serum of 10 normal volunteers resulted in 6.7, 7.8, 5.8, 9.7, 10.4, 6.6, 11.2, 6.9, 8.2, and 7.7 μg/dl. Find (a) the arithmetic mean, (b) the sample standard deviation, and (c) the 95% confidence range.
8. Can any of the observations of Problem 7 be rejected?
9. A well-type scintillation counter yields 1 million c/min/μCi using a standard of ^{131}I. Under the same counting conditions, background measures 800 c/4 min. What is the MDA for ^{131}I?
10. Two counts made with a long-lived source resulted in 2478 c/4 min and 3634 c/6 min. Is the detector operating properly?

REFERENCES

Bernier, D.R., Christian, P.E., and Langan, J.K., *Nuclear Medicine Technology & Techniques*, 3d ed., Mosby, St. Louis, 1994.

Bethge, K. et al., *Medical Applications of Nuclear Physics*, Springer–Verlag, Berlin, 2004.

Bevalacqua, J.J., *Basic Health Physics — Problems and Solutions*, Wiley–VCH, Weinheim, Germany, 1999.

Brogsitter, C. et al., ^{18}F-FDG PET for detecting myocardial viability: Validation of 3D data acquisition, *J. Nucl. Med.* 46, 19, 2005.

Code of Federal Regulations, Title 10, National Archives and Records Administration, Washington, DC, 2005.

Dowd, S.B. and Tilson, E.R., *Practical Radiation Protection and Applied Radiobiology*, 2d ed., Saunders, 1999.

Early, P.J. and Sodee, D.B., *Principles and Practice of Nuclear Medicine*, 2d ed., Mosby, St. Louis, MO, 1995.

Fiola, C., Monoclonal antibodies as anticancer agents, *U.S. Pharmacist*, 28, 10, 2003.

Israel, O. et al., Combined functional and structural evaluation of cancer patients with a hybrid camera-based PET/CT system using ^{18}F-FDG, *J. Nucl. Med.* 43, 1129, 2002.

Klingensmith, W.C., Eshima, D., and Goddard, J., *Nuclear Medicine Procedure Manual*, Oxford Medical, Englewood, NJ, 1991.

Lartizien, C. et al., A lesion detection observer study comparing 2-dimensional versus fully 3-dimensional whole-body PET imaging protocols, *J. Nucl. Med.* 45, 4714, 2004.

Love, C. and Palestro, C.J., Radionuclide imaging of infection, *J.Nucl. Med. Technol.* 32, 47, 2004.

Nabi, H.A. and Zubeldia, J.M., Clinical applications of ^{18}F-FDG in oncology, *J. Nucl. Med. Technol.* 30, 3, 2002.

Noz, M.E. and Maguire, G.Q., *Radiation Protection in the Radiologic and Health Sciences*, 2d ed., Lea & Febiger, Philadelphia, 1985.

Radiological Health Handbook, U.S. Department of Health, Education, and Welfare, Rockville, 1970.

Roberts, E.G. and Shulkin, B.L., Technical issues in performing PET studies in pediatric patients, *J. Nucl. Med. Technol.* 32, 5, 2004.

Saha, G.B., *Physics and Radiobiology of Nuclear Medicine*, Springer–Verlag, New York, 1993.

Saha, G.B., *Basics of PET imaging*, Springer, New York, 2005.

Shleien, B., Slaback, Jr., L.A., and Birky, B.K., *Handbook of Health Physics and Radiological Health*, 3d ed., Lippincott Williams & Wilkins, Philadelphia, 1998.

Sorenson, J.A. and Phelps, M E., *Physics in Nuclear Medicine*, 2d ed., W.B. Saunders, Philadelphia, 1987.

Steves, A.M., *Review of Nuclear Medicine Technology*, 2d ed., Society of Nuclear Medicine, Reston, VA, 1996.

Townsend, D.W. et al., PET/CT today and tomorrow, *J. Nucl. Med.* 45, 4S, 2004.

Zimmerman, B.E. and Pipes, D.W., Experimental determination of dose calibrator settings and study of associated volume dependence in V-vials for rhenium-186 perrhenate solution sources, *J. Nucl. Med.* 28, 264, 2000.

Zubal, I.G., Merging the instrumentation evolution, *J. Nucl. Med.* 42, 633, 2001.

5 Radiation Safety in the Nuclear Medicine Department

I. RATIONALE

The most important component of radiation safety is knowledge. NMTs and students of nuclear medicine technology must learn quickly that, to practice safety, they need to familiarize themselves with everything that is being done in the NM department. The NM department serves the community by providing (a) diagnostic procedures, mostly imaging, that depict functional images of the patients' organ systems and (b) therapeutic radionuclide procedures that alleviate the patients' illnesses. Furthermore, the staff of the NM department must perform their work while abiding by strict federal laws, state regulations, and in-house administrative policies.

Diagnostic procedures involve ordering of the prescribed RPs, the use of nuclide generators and kits to prepare RPs, the QA (quality assurance) testing of RPs, the assaying of unit and multiple dosage RPs using dose calibrators, the interviewing of patients, the dispensing of dosages of RPs for patients, the verification of dosages, the administration of RPs to patients, the QA of imaging instrumentation, the performance of the procedures themselves by planar, SPECT, or PET imaging, and the delivery of images to the physicians for proper interpretation.

Radionuclide therapy procedures involve the ordering of the prescribed therapeutic agents, the interviewing of patients, the providing of written instructions to patients, the preparation of the patients' rooms, the dispensing of the patients' dosages, the adhering to a very strict protocol during and after the administration of the therapeutic agent, the monitoring of patients' bodies and rooms at scheduled times, and the decontamination of the rooms at the conclusion of the patients' hospitalization.

Radiation safety is the common denominator of all procedures. Radiation workers are responsible for their own safety, that of other workers, including the clerical staff, and that of visitors. They must comply not only with the safety rules of the hospital's radiation safety program but with the practice of ALARA.

In this chapter, a basic design of an NM department and a brief description of the tasks performed are presented and discussed. This is followed by an introduction to the daily practice of radiation safety.

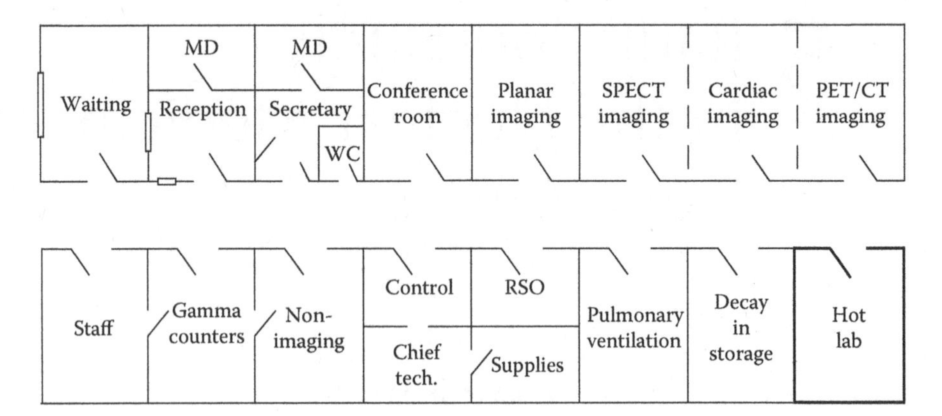

FIGURE 5.1 Basic design of an NM department. Cold areas are near the entrance on the left; warm areas and hot areas are toward the right.

II. DESIGN OF THE NM DEPARTMENT

The physical facilities of an NM department must ensure an efficient, safe, and economical operation. The design depends on the patient load and type of operation. In this section, the basic design of an NM department is described. The NM department works closely with the departments of radiology, medical sonography, and magnetic resonance imaging (MRI). In some medical centers, all these departments form a single imaging division.

The design of a typical, medium-size NM department is shown in Figure 5.1. For instructional purposes, we can tour the department from left to right, according to the levels of radioactivity handled in the various sections.

A. Cold Areas

These are the areas open to the public, clerical employees, and visitors. No radioactivity is handled in these areas. No radioactive packages or sources are brought into this area, and no radioactive patients are asked to wait there. These areas are the waiting room, the reception room, and the clerical offices. They are also referred to as nonrestricted areas. The exposure level must never exceed 2 mR/h (20 μSv/h) and 100 mrem/y (1 mSv/y). In other words, exposure rates should always be at background exposure levels. Although located within a restricted area, the physicians' offices, the staff lounge, the chief technologist's office, the control room, and the conference room are also areas in which no radioactivity is handled and, in the spirit of ALARA, should also be cold areas.

B. Lukewarm Areas

These are areas in which very low levels of radioactivity are handled, usually microcurie (kBq) levels only. Examples are the nonimaging procedures room and the gamma counters room (thyroid uptakes, Schilling tests, blood radioassays, wipe/swab-tests).

C. Warm Areas

In these areas, millicurie (MBq) levels of radioactivity are handled daily. Examples are the imaging rooms, including the pulmonary ventilation room and the PET/CT room. In these rooms, some procedures may require only 0.3 mCi (11.1 MBq), and other procedures may require 30 mCi (1.11 GBq) of a radiopharmaceutical.

D. Hot Areas

From 1 mCi (37 MBq) to 1 Ci (37 GBq) may be handled in shielded containers and enclosures or stored in shielded cabinets in "hot areas." Examples are the radiopharmacy or "hot lab" and the "decay-in-storage" areas. The radiopharmacy or hot lab is where radiopharmaceuticals are prepared or received in multiple dose vials, quality-assurance tested, and dispensed into individual dosages. The decay-in-storage room is possibly located in a remote area of the hospital. This area is where radioactive waste is allowed to decay to background levels before disposal. See Chapter 7.

III. DESCRIPTION OF SOME AREAS

A. Waiting Room and Reception

As outpatients (referrals) arrive, they check in with the receptionist. The control room is alerted, and the preparation for the NM procedure starts. The reception and waiting rooms are nonrestricted areas. Exposure rates do not exceed 2 mrem/h (20 μSv/h). Inpatients (hospitalized) are brought to the NM department as scheduled. They check in with the receptionist and go to the assigned area.

B. Nonimaging Procedures Room

Tests that require very low levels of radioactivity are performed in this room. Examples are radioimmunoassays (RIAs), the thyroid uptake of radioiodide, the vitamin B_{12} absorption test (Schilling test), and the blood volume determinations. See Table 5.1.

TABLE 5.1
Diagnostic Nonimaging Procedures

Procedure	Radiotracer
Schilling test	^{57}Co-vitamin B_{12}
Blood/plasma volumes	^{125}I-human serum albumin
Platelet survival	^{111}In-autologous platelets
RBC mass/survival	^{51}Cr-chromate
Test for *Helicobacter pylori*	^{14}C-urea
Thyroid uptake	^{131}I-iodide, ^{123}I-iodide
Ferro- and erythrokinetics	^{59}Fe-citrate, ^{51}Cr-chromate

1. Radioimmunoassays (RIAs)

Patients requiring "blood work" are led to this room for obtaining a blood sample so that the prescribed *in vitro* tests (RIAs) can be ordered and performed. These tests may be done in other sections of the hospital because they involve exempt quantities of radioactivity. They measure minute concentrations of hormones, drugs, or metabolic substances in the patient's blood serum or plasma.

2. Thyroid Uptake of Radioiodide

A basic step in the study of thyroid gland physiology is the uptake of iodide. In NM, this step is studied using radioactive ^{131}I-iodide or ^{123}I-iodide. The patient returns for a measurement of the radioactivity in the thyroid gland from 6 to 24 h later using an external scintillation detector or a gamma camera. The activity found and its distribution are an expression of the physiopathology of the thyroid gland. If ^{123}I is used, thyroid gland imaging follows. In any case, the technologist records all results on a special form and hands it over, along with the images, to the physician for interpretation.

3. Schilling Test

In this test, the patient receives a trace dosage of ^{57}Co-vitamin B_{12}, and the radioactivity excreted with the urine at 24 h is measured to reflect the absorption of the vitamin through the GI tract. Results are reported to the physician for interpretation.

4. Blood Volume Test

A trace amount of ^{125}I-human serum albumin is given intravenously to the patient. A few minutes later, one or more blood samples are drawn. The radioactivity is measured and the radioactivity concentration is calculated. From this concentration, the blood volume is determined. Using the packed cell volume (PCV) test, the plasma volume and the total red cell volume can be calculated. Results are taken to the physician for interpretation.

C. Control Room

The technologist assigned to this area is responsible for the timely scheduling of patients, procedures, and staff assignments. In the event of emergency scans or cancellations, the control room technologist makes adjustments to continue the uninterrupted operation of the department.

D. Imaging Rooms

For most procedures, planar, SPECT, or PET imaging, technologists bring the prescribed doses of RPs in shielded syringes placed inside shielded containers from the hot lab to the assigned imaging rooms, where patients are already positioned on an imaging table and ready. When all preparations are completed, the RP is injected intravenously. The imaging data acquisition can begin immediately. Some patients

TABLE 5.2
Technetium-99m Imaging Procedures

Procedure	Imaging Agent
Acute infections	^{99m}Tc-Autologous WBCs
Appendicitis	^{99m}Tc-Lanolesomab
Brain SPECT	^{99m}Tc-HMPAO
Breast imaging	^{99m}Tc-Sestamibi
Cardiac ventriculography	^{99m}Tc-Teboroxime
Colorectal tumors	^{99m}Tc-CEA
Cystogram	^{99m}Tc-Pertechnetate
Deep vein thrombosis	^{99m}Tc-Apcitide, ^{99m}Tc-FBD
Gastric emptying	^{99m}Tc-S-Colloid Meal
GI bleeding	^{99m}Tc-Pyrophosphate-RBCs
Hepatobiliary	^{99m}Tc-Disofenin/Mebrofenin
Liver hemangioma	^{99m}Tc-Pyrophosphate-RBCs
Liver/spleen	^{99m}Tc-S-Colloid
Lung perfusion	^{99m}Tc-MAA
Lung ventilation	^{99m}Tc-DTPA aerosol
Lung malignancies	^{99m}Tc-Depreotide
Lymphoscintigraphy	^{99m}Tc-S-Colloid (<0.22 μm)
Meckel's diverticulum	^{99m}Tc-Pertechnetate
Melanoma	^{99m}Tc-Interleukin-2
Myocardial infarction	^{99m}Tc-Glucarate
Myocardial SPECT	^{99m}Tc-MIBI, ^{99m}Tc-Tetrophosmin
Osteomyelitis	^{99m}Tc-Interleukin-8
Parathyroid	^{99m}Tc-MIBI
Renal cortex	^{99m}Tc-DMSA, ^{99m}Tc-GH
Renal GFR	^{99m}Tc-DTPA
Renal tubular function	^{99m}Tc-MAG3
Skeletal	^{99m}Tc-MDP, ^{99m}Tc-HDP
Testicular	^{99m}Tc-Pertechnetate
Thyroid	^{99m}Tc-Pertechnetate

are injected in their hospital rooms and later are brought to the NM department for imaging. In the pulmonary ventilation room, ^{133}Xe gas or ^{99m}Tc-DTPA aerosol is administered by inhalation using a specially designed dispenser. In all imaging rooms, technologists are responsible for the good care of patients, the radiation safety of the patients and the staff, as well as the quality assurance of the imaging instrumentation. Table 5.2 and Table 5.3 list some diagnostic imaging procedures and the RPs used.

E. Radiopharmacy (Hot Lab)

This is the room where the highest levels of radioactivity are handled. Some of the tasks performed there are (a) reception of generators and RPs, (b) monitoring of all packages containing radioactivities, (c) logging of all radioactivities upon arrival,

TABLE 5.3
Other Radionuclides Imaging Procedures

Procedure	Imaging Agent
Acute infections	Autologous ^{111}In-WBCs
Adrenal cortex	^{131}I-NP59
Adrenal medulla	^{131}I-MIBI
Brain PET	^{18}F-FDG, ^{18}F-Fluorodopa
Breast	^{125}I-B72.3 MAb
Cardiac ventriculography	^{82}Rb-chloride, ^{15}O-water
Chronic infections, tumors	^{67}Ga-citrate
Cisternography	^{111}In-DTPA
Colorectal tumors	^{111}In-Satumomab pendetide, ^{125}I-B72.3 MAb
Lung perfusion	^{15}O-water
Lung ventilation	^{133}Xe-gas
Myocardial infarction	^{111}In-anti-myosin Ab
Myocardial SPECT	^{201}Tl-Thallous chloride
Myocardial PET	^{18}F-FDG, ^{82}Rb-chloride
Neuroendocrine tumors	^{111}In-Pentetreotide
Non-Hodgkins lymphoma	^{111}In-Ibritumomab
Ovarian malignancy	^{111}In-Satumomab pendetide
Parathyroid	^{201}Tl-Thallous chloride
Prostatic cancer	^{111}In-Capromab, ^{11}C-methionine
Thyroid	^{123}I-iodide
Tumors, PET	^{18}F-FDG

(d) preparation and/or dispensing of dosages of RPs for patients, (e) elution and QA of dose calibrators, (f) lab monitorings, and (g) record keeping of all of the foregoing. Figure 5.2 shows a section of the hot lab. Notice a glove box, a dose calibrator, shielding cabinets for storage, and a lavatory. Figure 5.3 shows a radiopharmacist drawing a dosage of an RP behind lead–glass shielding. Figure 5.4 shows a lead container for storage of radioactive sources. Figure 5.5 shows shields for multidose vials and a tungsten syringe shield for injections of RPs. Figure 5.6 shows a pocket bleeper radiation monitor ideal for radiopharmacists and NMTs working in the hot areas of the NM department. All those shielding devices and dosimeters are extremely useful in maintaining a safe environment and minimizing personnel exposures.

IV. MOLECULAR MEDICINE

Nuclear medicine is in a unique position in the new emerging field of molecular medicine. The use of radiotracers that bind specific target molecules (molecular targeting) in diseased cells or tissues has been a method of localization used in NM for many years. The radiotracer binds a mutated locus in DNA, or its related RNAs,

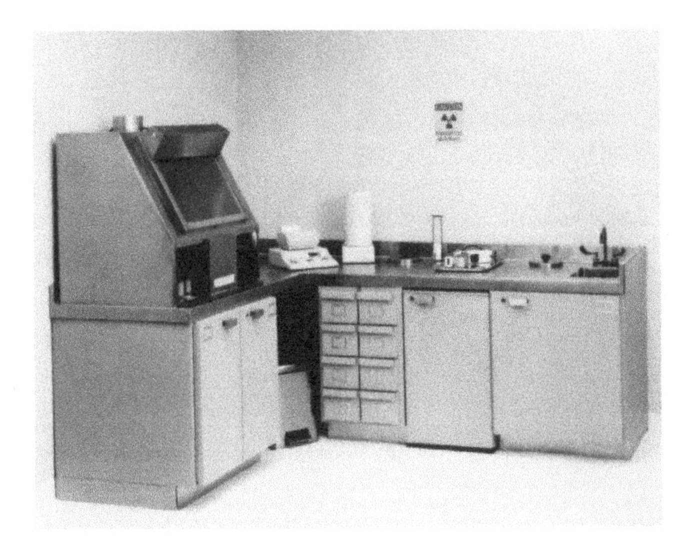

FIGURE 5.2 A view of the radiopharmacy or hot lab. A glove box appears on the left, a dose calibrator on the center, and a lavatory on the right. There are shielded cabinets and shielded drawers under the counters. (Courtesy of Fluke Biomedical, Cleveland, OH.)

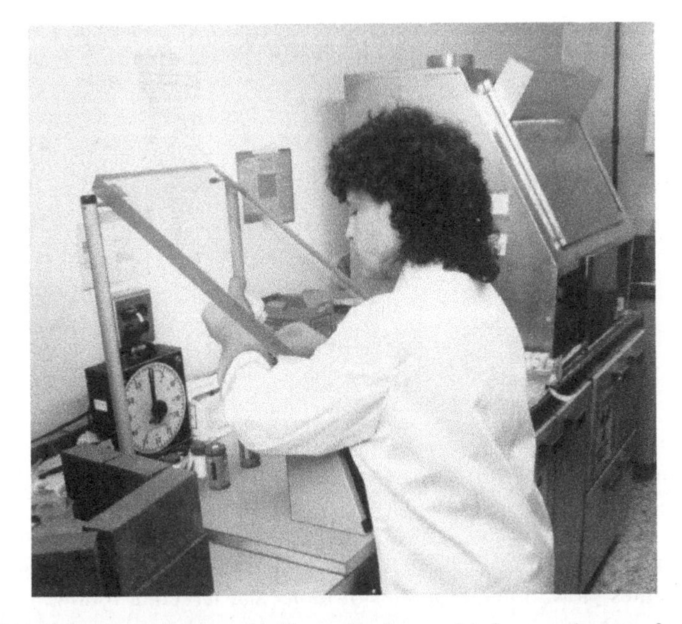

FIGURE 5.3 Behind a lead–glass shield, a radiopharmacist draws a dosage of a radiopharmaceutical for a patient. (Courtesy of Fluke Biomedical, Cleveland, OH.)

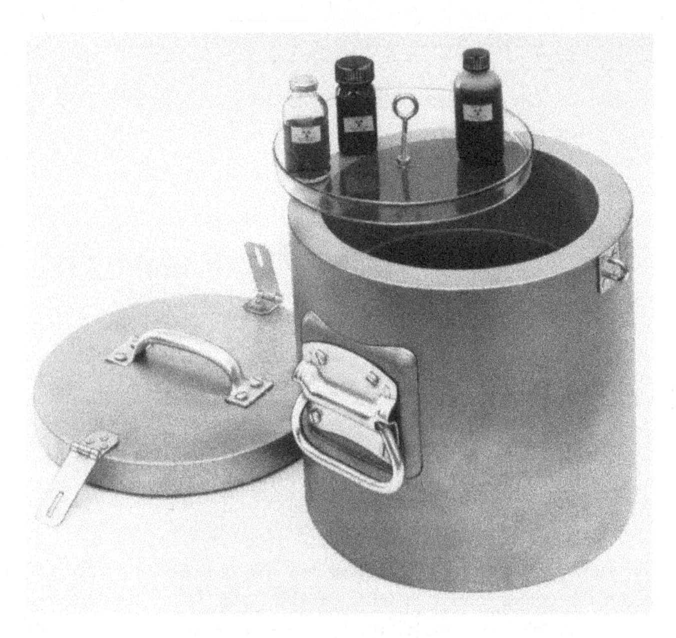

FIGURE 5.4 Heavy shielded container used for storage of radioactive standards and other sources. (Courtesy of Fluke Biomedical, Cleveland, OH.)

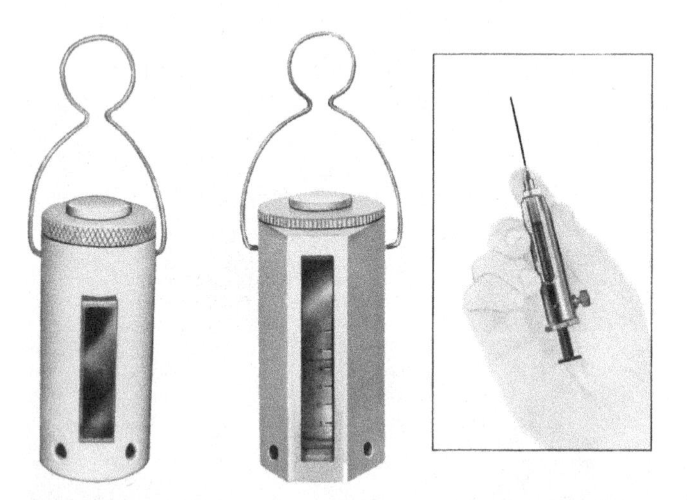

FIGURE 5.5 Two lead shielding devices for multidosage vials (left) and a tungsten shield for hypodermic syringes (right). All items shown have lead–glass windows. (Courtesy of Fluke Biomedical, Cleveland, OH.)

or their protein products. Under the SPECT camera or the PET/CT scanner, the target molecules glow. Some examples of molecular targeting follow.

1. ^{99m}Tc-CD15 is a monoclonal antibody (MAb) that targets a specific antigen in neutrophils. The imaging procedure is indicated in osteomyelitis,

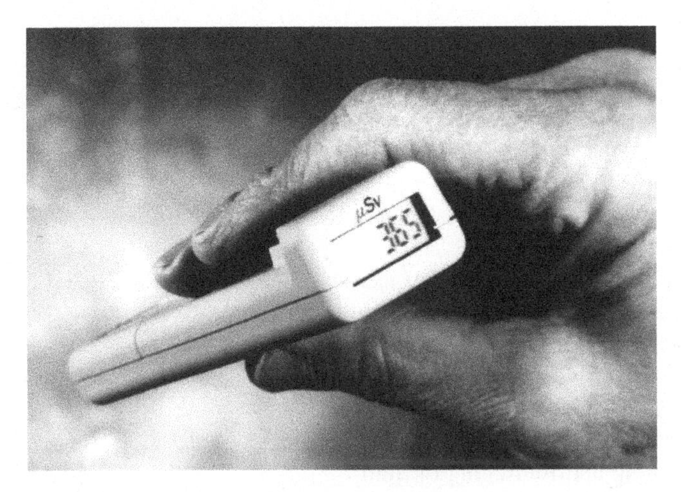

FIGURE 5.6 A personal bleeper radiation monitor. Bleep rates: Background: 1 bleep/15–30 min; 1 mR/h: 1 bleep/20 s; 100 mR/h: continuous alarm signal. (Courtesy of Fluke Biomedical, Cleveland, OH.)

fever of unknown origin (FUO), post-surgical abscesses, inflammatory bowel disease, and in pulmonary illnesses.

2. ^{18}F-FDG (fluorodeoxyglucose) is a marker of glucose transport expression. This radiotracer concentrates in normal or abnormal tissues in proportion to their metabolic rate. The imaging procedure is indicated in tumor detection, evaluation of cancer therapy, myocardial viability, and hypometabolism in mental illnesses.
3. ^{111}In-octreotide targets somatostatin receptors in neuroendocrine tumors; ^{99m}Tc-depreotide targets somatostatin receptors in carcinomas of the lungs.
4. ^{131}I- and ^{123}I-MIBG (meta-iodobenzylguanidine) target normal epinephrine in phechromocytomas and neuroblastomas.
5. Antitumor monoclonal antibodies labeled with ^{111}In or ^{99m}Tc are used to target antigens in the diagnoses of malignant illnesses. Labeled with ^{131}I, ^{125}I, or ^{90}Y, MAbs are used in the therapy of those illnesses.

The specificity, sensitivity, and accuracy of nuclear medicine procedures are very much enhanced by the merging of PET and CT imaging. PET shows function, metabolism; CT shows exquisite anatomy of the targeted tissues. Molecular targeting is here to stay.

V. THE RADIATION SAFETY PROGRAM (RSP)

A. General Considerations

The RSP is a document concerned with the compliance with all the safety rules and regulations as they apply to the hospital or medical center (10CFR20.1105). Some specific rules are described in the hospital license. The RSO and the radiation safety committee are responsible for writing, editing, and approving those rules. The document in the final form is submitted to the licensing agency and is revised once a year to make adjustments concerning new procedures or changes in the staff.

B. Contents

The following items may be included in the RSP:

1. The Radioactive Materials License (10CFR30.31; 10CFR35.12)
2. The Radiation Safety Committee (RSC)
3. The Radiation Safety Officer (RSO)
4. The Quality Management Program (QMP)
5. The ALARA Program
6. Authorized Users of Radioactivity
7. Training and Retraining of Staff
8. Personnel Exposure Records
9. Record-Keeping
10. Inspections
11. Reception of Radioactive Packages
12. Radiopharmaceuticals
13. Dose Calibrators
14. Laboratory Rules
15. Use of Radioactive Materials
16. Radioactive Waste Disposal
17. Laboratory Surveys
18. Radiation Emergencies

VI. RADIATION SAFETY COMMITTEE (RSC)

The RSC plays an important role in the planning and maintaining of a safe operation in the hospital. The RSO is the secretary of the committee. He or she prepares the agenda for the committee meetings, which are held quarterly or more often if needed. Other members are a representative from the administration, the medical director, a representative from nursing, the chief technologist, the radiopharmacist, and other authorized users. The committee approves changes or revisions to the RSP before submission to the licensing agency, makes sure that all new procedures are safe, and ensures the practice of radiation safety and ALARA at all times.

VII. RADIATION SAFETY OFFICER (RSO)

The licensee appoints a qualified person to perform the duties of RSO. The RSO is the person responsible for the implementation of the RSP. The licensee's administration must give the RSO authority and support in the performance of his/her duties (10CFR35.50). In addition to participation in the RSC, the RSO does the following:

1. Investigates and reports all radiation safety incidents (10CFR20.2202); personnel overexposures; losses of radioactive sources (10CFR20.2201); transfers of radioactive sources; and RP misadministrations. The RSO reports to the RSC and prescribes corrective action.
2. Prepares written policies on purchase of RPs; the receiving of radioactive packages (10CFR20.1906); and the storage, use, and disposal of radioactive materials. In addition, the RSO posts radiation warning signs where appropriate (10CFR20.1901).
3. Writes policies on radiation emergencies, and directs corrective action during emergencies.
4. Manages and maintains records of the staff radiation exposures (10CFR20.2106).
5. Prepares written procedures on radiation surveys, schedules surveys, and ensures records of surveys are maintained (10CFR20.1501,1502).
6. Prepares written procedures for radioactive waste disposal (10CFR20.2001).
7. Provides training to new personnel. As needed, provides retraining of all staff.
8. Prepares and implements an ALARA program (see below).
9. Organizes and participates actively in all RSC meetings.
10. With the RSC, prepares a QMP (10CFR35.40).

VIII. RADIOACTIVE MATERIALS LICENSE

The radioactive materials license is a document issued by the NRC or the licensing agency in agreement states. The license authorizes the licensee to own and use by-product materials (10CFR35.13). In agreement states, it might also concern accelerator-produced radioactive compounds. The license recognizes authorized users and their supervision of other staff, lists the authorized radionuclides and the quantities allowed, and also gives the special conditions under which those materials can be used. The license is normally renewed every five years. The license can be amended as needed at any time following a written request by the licensee (10CFR35.13).

IX. QUALITY MANAGEMENT PROGRAM (QMP)

A. Definition

The QMP is a document submitted to the licensing agency. The QMP ensures that the licensee follows specific requirements:

1. Will not administer RPs to humans without a written directive.
2. Will abide by the prescribed directives.
3. Will maintain records of all RP administrations.
4. Will revise the QMP annually.
5. Will take appropriate action when a misadministration or a recordable event occurs.

B. Misadministrations

Misadministrations apply to by-product material only. They fall in three categories:

1. Diagnostic radioiodine: only for dosages of ^{131}I or ^{125}I in quantities of less than 30 μCi (1.11 MBq), administration to the wrong patient, administration of the wrong RP, giving the wrong dosage increased by more than 20% of the prescribed dose, and the difference being greater than 30 μCi.
2. Other diagnostic RPs, including ^{99m}Tc: wrong patient, wrong RP, wrong dosage, wrong route of administration, and the resulting deep dose to the patient is greater than 5 rem (50 μSv) or the organ dose is greater than 50 rem (500 μSv).
3. Therapeutic: dosing the wrong patient, administering the wrong RP, administering the wrong dosage, using the wrong route of administration, and giving a dose greater than the prescribed dose by more than 20%.

C. Recordable Events

Events that must be entered in the record files but do not need to be reported to the licensing agency:

1. Diagnostic: only for ^{131}INa and ^{125}INa dosages greater than 30 μCi (1.11 MBq), administration of an RP without a written directive, no record of a written directive, the dosage differs by more than 10% and the difference is greater than 15 μCi (555 kBq).
2. Therapeutic: for any therapeutic radiopharmaceutical, no written directive, no record of a written directive, and the dosage differs by more than 10%.

D. Reportable Events

All misadministrations must be reported to the licensing agency according to the following procedure:

1. Within 24 h of the event: by telephone to the licensing agency, to the referring physician, and to the parent or guardian if the patient is a minor.
2. Within 15 d: written report to the licensing agency, to the referring physician, to the parent or guardian if the patient is a minor. The QMP filed with the licensing agency must include a plan to prevent future similar events.
3. Records must be kept for 5 years.

X. THE ALARA PROGRAM

A. Objective

The licensee must develop and implement a written ALARA program aimed at minimizing exposures reasonably. With the support of the administration, the RSO enforces ALARA. The program may include

1. Notices to radiation workers about the RSP
2. Statement of ALARA warning levels (10% of dose limits)
3. Statement of ALARA action levels (30% of dose limits)
4. Policy regarding pregnant workers
5. Safe-handling procedures
6. Procedures for ensuring the staff's continuing education
7. Procedures for training and retraining of the staff

1. Inclusion

The ALARA program can be included in the RSP submitted yearly to the licensing agency.

XI. THE PRACTICE OF RADIATION SAFETY

A. Authorized Users

Authorized users are persons responsible for compliance with the terms of the license. Their names appear in the license. Usually, nuclear physicians and radiopharmacists are the authorized users. They may supervise technologists and other radiation workers, who, in turn, are also certified and licensed to handle radioactive materials. Any change in the authorized users list requires an amendment to the license.

B. Training of Personnel

All medical radiation workers in the United States must demonstrate competency by passing a National Certification Board Exam. In addition, in many states, workers must be licensed by the licensing agency. To renew the license, they must demonstrate having earned current continuing education (CE) credits. Those who were trained more than seven years earlier must be retrained. In 2003, the Society of Nuclear Medicine, technology section, recommended that NMTs must get additional training and demonstrate competency to operate PET/CT scanners.

C. Personnel Exposures

All radiation workers in the NM department likely to receive 10% of the occupational dose limits must be continuously monitored for whole-body exposure. Records of personnel exposure must be kept indefinitely. For workers transferring from one institution to another, an effort must be made to obtain the previous exposure records (10CFR20.1501).

D. Record Keeping

Licensing agencies require that some activities be performed on a specific schedule and that records of such activities be kept for some specified length of time. An outline of record-keeping times follows:

1. Three years: audits of the RSP, reports of exposure history, receipt or transfer of radioactive materials, QMP reviews, recordable events, dose calibrators QA tests, calibration of survey meters, assay of patient doses, area surveys, release of patients, decay in storage, ^{99}Mo breakthroughs, and therapy patient surveys.
2. Five years: misadministrations, inventory of sealed sources, and leak testings of sealed sources.
3. Duration of use: dose calibrator geometry corrections, manufacturer's sealed sources instructions, and radioactive gases calculations.
4. Duration of the license: radiation safety program, personnel exposure monitoring, disposal of radioactivities, minutes of the RSC meetings, and bioassays.

E. Inspections (10CFR19.14, 10CFR30.52)

The licensing agency can inspect the medical facilities, materials, and records at reasonable times to verify compliance with the license. Inspectors may speak privately with workers. The RSO or another designated person should assist the inspectors with the examination of records. Inspections might last 8 h and end with an exit interview with the appropriate administrator to discuss the findings. A letter from the licensing agency to the administrator will follow indicating the points of noncompliance, if any. The licensee will have 30 d to respond and to state the corrective action and the time of implementation of such corrective action. If full compliance is found, this information will be included in the letter, and no reply will be required.

F. Reception of Radioactive Packages

Reception of such packages is regulated by the licensing agency (10CFR20.1906). Local regulations must be consulted. External monitoring of packages must be done within 3 h of their arrival. Exposure rates must not exceed those for categories I, II, or III, listed in Table 3.1. Wipe-testing, if required, must not exceed 2200 DPM/100 cm^2. For PET RPs, wipe-tests must not exceed 22,000 DPM/100 cm^2. By knowing the efficiency of the radiation detector, the DPMs can be calculated as follows:

$$\text{DPM} = \text{CPM}/\text{Counter Efficiency}$$

The counter efficiency is determined by counting a standard (known DPMs) under specific geometric conditions:

$$\text{Counter Efficiency} = \text{Net CPM}/\text{Standard DPM}$$

Records of package monitorings and wipe testings must be kept for three years. Packages that exceed the specified exposure rates must be reported to the delivery carrier and to the licensing agency.

G. Radiopharmaceuticals

Handling RPs and other radioactive sources depends largely on the type and magnitude of the NM practice. For instructional purposes, medical centers, hospitals, and clinics may be grouped into one of the following categories:

1. PET centers: These centers are large medical institutions with a hospital and a cyclotron facility. They have the professional staff to operate the cyclotron and the chemical synthesizers. They produce the positron emitting radionuclides and PET compounds needed for in-house imaging as well as for supplying other hospitals and clinics within a large metropolitan area. In these facilities, because of their short half-lives, PET radiopharmaceuticals are tested "after-the-fact," meaning at a later time with the charge of reporting and recording the results properly. Table 4.3 and Table 4.4 list the positron emitters and the PET RPs produced and used in PET centers.
2. Medium-sized hospitals: These institutions may have 400–500 beds and a large NM department. They have a full-time pharmacist and a full-time RSO. They prepare daily a large spectrum of RPs and they can even provide RPs to other hospitals. They may use one or two ^{99m}Tc generators per week. They usually purchase accelerator-produced RPs from regional RP companies for PET and other imaging procedures. Table 5.2 lists the most common imaging procedures using ^{99m}Tc compounds, and Table 5.3 shows the imaging procedures using other radionuclide imaging agents.
3. Small hospitals and clinics: These centers may have a small radiopharmacy and a part-time radiopharmacist. They use one ^{99m}Tc generator per week. They prepare routine RPs using commercial kits and QA-test them daily. NM technologists are trained to prepare RPs and to do imaging of patients during periods when they are on call (nights or weekends). Other RPs are purchased from regional radiopharmacies or PET centers.

H. Dose Calibrators

Dose calibrators are extremely useful in the radiopharmacy or hot lab. All generator eluants, RPs, and patient dosages are measured with the dose calibrator. Most NM departments need at least two. As required by the licensing agency, dose calibrators must be QA-tested at regular intervals. Briefly, QA tests include the following:

1. *Constancy* (precision, reproducibility): Done daily using a long-lived standard. Readings must stay within 10% of the mean.
2. *Accuracy*: Done at installation, then annually. Three standards are used. Readings cannot differ by more than 10% from the certified activity.
3. *Linearity* (decay of ^{99m}Tc): Done at installation, then quarterly. Calculated decay values and measured decay values of a ^{99m}Tc source must agree

within 10%. Approved linearity kits that simulate decay accurately can be used to perform the test in a short time.

4. *Geometry*: Done at installation. If different configurations (syringe and vial sizes) differ by more than 10%, correcting factors must be determined and used.

I. Laboratory Rules

Rules are essential to radiation safety. Please refer to Chapter 6.

J. Use of Radioactive Materials

Only licensed institutions and their staff can use radioactive materials. Authorized users can supervise other workers in the use of such materials. Some special rules are as follows:

1. Users shall handle radioactive gases and aerosols in such a manner that airborne radioactivities do not exceed the set limits. (See Chapter 3.) Disposal of those gases or aerosols must follow proper procedures.
2. Each elution from a ^{99m}Tc generator must be assayed for ^{99m}Tc and for ^{99}Mo breakthrough (10CFR35.204). At the time of injection, the latter must not exceed 0.15 μCi of ^{99}Mo per millicurie of ^{99m}Tc (0.15 kBq of ^{99}Mo per MBq of ^{99m}Tc). In the eluant, ^{99m}Tc is decaying faster than ^{99}Mo. Therefore, the concentration of ^{99}Mo relative to that of ^{99m}Tc increases with time.

   Then, a logical question is: How long before an eluant reaches the 0.15 μCi/mCi limit? Figure 5.7 and Table 5.4 provide the answers. The equation is

$$\mu Ci/mCi = 0.15e^{-0.105t} \tag{5.1}$$

3. Eluates must also be assayed for aluminum breakthrough. The generator supplier usually provides the customer with a colorimetric kit for this purpose. The limit is 10 μg of aluminum per ml of eluate.
4. Persons eluting generators, preparing RPs, performing QA of RPs, and dispensing patient doses must wear a hand or ring dosimeter. Elution records must be kept for three years.
5. All RPs must be stored in shielded refrigerators or shielded cabinets while not in use.

K. Radioactive Waste Disposal

See also Chapter 7. Some basic rules are as follows(10CFR20.2001):

1. For radionuclides with half-lives shorter than 120 d, wastes can be allowed to decay in storage (DIS) before disposal with the nonradioactive waste

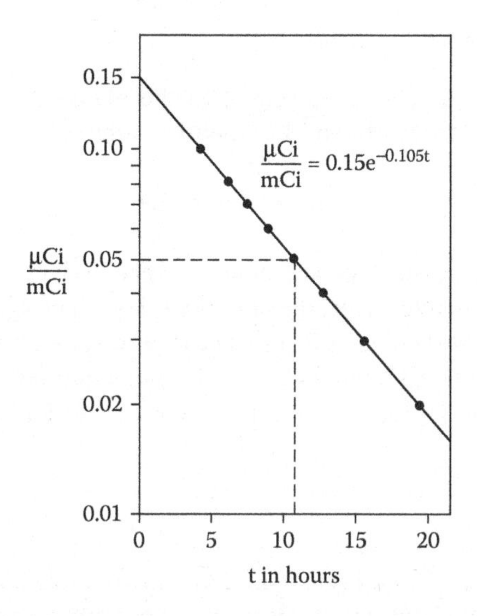

FIGURE 5.7 Time in which ^{99m}Tc eluants reach the ^{99}Mo breakthrough limit. Select the μCi/mCi on the ordinate. Go to the curve, and follow the abscissa to read *t*, the time to reach the limit. On the top right is the equation that describes the ratio–time relationship.

TABLE 5.4
Time for ^{99m}Tc Eluants to Reach the ^{99}Mo Breakthrough Limit

μCi/mCi	Time
0.14	40 min
0.13	1 h + 22 min
0.12	2 h + 8 min
0.11	2 h + 57 min
0.10	3 h + 52 min
0.09	4 h + 52 min
0.08	5 h + 59 min
0.07	7 h + 15 min
0.06	8 h + 42 min
0.05	10 h + 30 min

(10CFR35.92). Most diagnostic and therapeutic radiopharmaceuticals fall in this category. They could also be disposed of through a licensed contractor.

2. Small amounts of radioactive solutions can be released into the sanitary sewer provided the monthly average concentration does not exceed specific concentration limits (10CFR20.2003); see Chapter 7.
3. Radioactive gases such as ^{133}Xe and aerosols such as ^{99m}Tc-DTPA aerosol must be handled in closed systems.

L. Laboratory Surveys

Laboratory radiation surveys are essential to the maintenance of a safe working environment in the NM department. Detailed procedures are given in Chapter 7.

1. Survey instruments must be calibrated annually (10CFR20.1501, 10CFR35.61).
2. Laboratory wipe-surveys are done as specified in the license. To be considered negative, wipes must contain less than 2,200 DPM/100 cm^2 or less than 6,600 DPM/300 cm^2. These correspond, respectively, to less than 1 and 3 nCi (37 and 111 Bq) of removable radioactivity. For PET imaging agents, wipes must not exceed 22,000 DPM/100cm^2 (10 nCi or 370 Bq).

M. Sealed Sources

Some sealed sources are used in the NM department as standards, as markers, and as QA testing sources. Leak-testing is required for alpha sources greater than 10 μCi (370 kBq) and beta sources greater than 100 μCi (3.7 MBq). Sealed sources are to be leak-tested at 6-month intervals and records kept during the time of use of the sources. Testing can be done using the wipe technique or using cotton swabs. Swabs must show that they do not contain more than 5 nCi (185 Bq) of removable radioactivity. Figure 5.8 shows a kit used in the leak-testing of sealed sources. Sources that exceed 5 nCi (185 Bq) must be reported to the licensing agency within 5 d.

N. Radionuclide Therapy

Radionuclide therapy is a very special area of NM applications. The use of beta emitters in the treatment of malignant disease and in the alleviation of pain caused by bone metastases is extremely important to patients. Readers are referred to Chapter 6 for a description of those procedures.

O. Radiation Emergencies

The most likely emergencies that can occur in the NM department are radioactive spills. These invariably result in unnecessary exposures. For example, a spill in the hot lab could involve 500 mCi of ^{99m}Tc. That could result in an exposure rate of 7 mR/min at 30 cm from the center of the spill (70 μSv/min). A spill of a patient dosage in the imaging areas could involve 30 mCi of ^{99m}Tc. The exposure rate would be 0.4 mR/min at 30 cm from the center of the spill (4 μSv/min). A 15-mCi spill of ^{18}F-FDG in the PET imaging room could result in an exposure rate of 1.6 mR/min (16 μSv/min) at 30 cm from the center of the spill. These situations are considered "major spills." Under the direction of the RSO, the decontamination procedure must be done immediately. See Chapter 7.

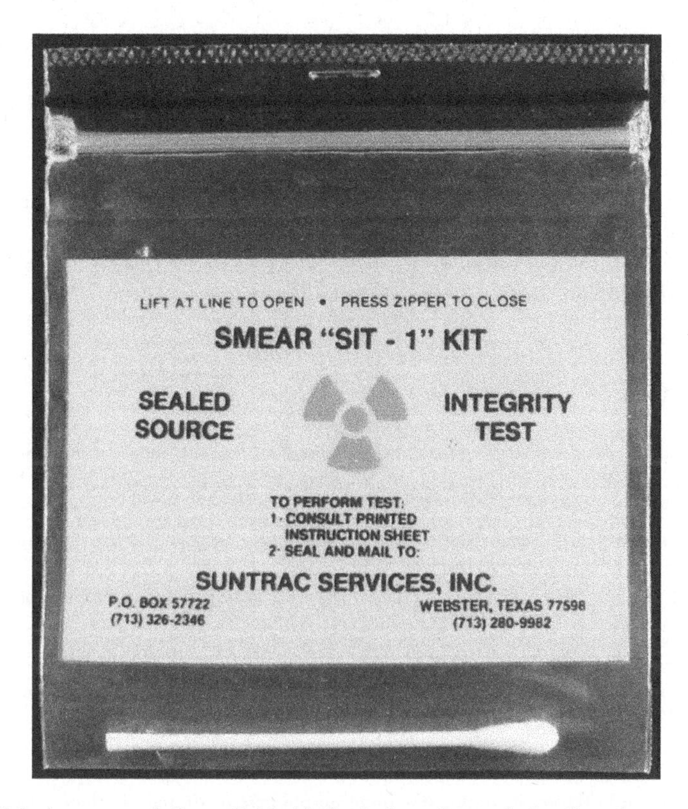

FIGURE 5.8 A commercially available kit for leak-testing sealed radioactive sources.

PROBLEMS

This problem set deals with patient dose calculations, an essential task performed many times daily in the NM department.

1. The concentration of an ^{123}I solution is 100 MBq/ml at 9:00 a.m. What volume will contain a dosage of 12 MBq at noon the next day?
2. A solution of ^{111}In-DTPA contains 150 MBq/ml on Tuesday at noon. What is its concentration 48 h later?
3. A vial of ^{133}Xe gas contains 400 MBq at 8:00 a.m. on Monday. What is its activity at 4:00 p.m. on Friday?
4. A patient receives 1 GBq of ^{131}I-iodide for treatment of hyperthyroidism. If his urine contains 0.6 GBq at 24 h, how much is left in his body?
5. We have 5 ml of a 1.6 GBq/ml ^{99m}Tc-pertechnetate solution. What volume of saline solution must we add to lower its concentration to 1.0 GBq/ml?
6. The concentration of a ^{201}Tl solution is 200 MBq/ml at 8:30 a.m. on Monday. What volume must we draw into a syringe on Tuesday at noon for a dosage of 100 MBq?

7. Some ^{123}I capsules contained 7.4 MBq each on Monday at noon. What is their activity at 8:00 a.m. on Friday?
8. A ^{99m}Tc generator arrives at 7:00 a.m. Monday containing 22 GBq of ^{99}Mo. If the generator is not used on Monday, how much ^{99m}Tc can we expect at 8:00 a.m. on Tuesday?
9. For any radionuclide, how many half-lives are needed for the activity to drop to 10, 1, and 0.1% of the original activity?
10. The activity of a source drops from 50 MBq to 35.3 MBq in 6.6 h. What is the half-life of the radionuclide?

REFERENCES

Bethge, K. et al., *Medical Applications of Nuclear Physics*, Springer–Verlag, Berlin, 2004.

Bevalacqua, J.J., *Basic Health Physics — Problems and Solutions*, Wiley–VCH, Weinheim, Germany, 1999.

Britz–Cunningham, S.H., and Adelstein, S.J., Molecular targeting with radionuclides: state of the science, *J. Nucl. Med.* 44, 1945, 2003.

Brogsitter, C. et al., ^{18}F-FDG PET for detecting myocardial viability: validation of 3D data acquisition, *J. Nucl. Med.* 46, 19, 2005.

Chandra, R., *Nuclear Medicine Physics — The Basics*, 6th ed., Lippincott Williams & Wilkins, Philadelphia, 2004.

Chilton, H.M. and Witcofski, R L., *Nuclear Pharmacy*, Lea & Febiger, Philadelphia, 1986.

Code of Federal Regulations, Title 10, National Archives and Records Administration, Washington, DC, 2005.

Conti, P.S., New horizons in molecular imaging-nuclear medicine, *J. Nucl. Med.*, 46, 14N, 2005.

Dowd, S.B. and Tilson, E.R., *Practical Radiation Protection and Applied Radiobiology*, 2d ed., Saunders, Philadelphia, 1999.

Early, P.J. and Sodee, D.B., *Principles and Practice of Nuclear Medicine*, 2d ed., Mosby, St. Louis, 1995.

Even-Sapir, E. et al., Role of ^{18}F-FDG dual-head gamma camera coincidence imaging in recurrent or metastatic colorectal carcinoma, *J. Nucl. Med.*, 43, 603, 2002.

ICRP, *Protection of the Patient in Nuclear Medicine*, Pergamon Press, Oxford, U.K., 1993.

Indium-111-Pentetreotide, package insert, Mallinckrodt, St. Louis, 2000.

Iodine-123-Meta-Iodobenzylguanidine, package insert, Nordion International, Inc., Torrance, 2002.

Israel, O. et al., Combined functional and structural evaluation of cancer patients with a hybrid camera-based PET/CT system using ^{18}F-FDG, *J. Nucl. Med.*, 43, 1129, 2002.

Kowalsky, R.J. and Falen, S.W., *Radiopharmaceuticals in Nuclear Pharmacy and Nuclear Medicine*, 2d ed., American Pharmacists Association, Washington, DC, 2004.

Mason, J.S., Elliott, K.M., and Mitro, A.C., *The Nuclear Medicne Handbbok for Achieving Compliance with NRC Regulations*, Society of Nuclear Medicine, Reston, VA, 1997.

NCRP Report 91: *Recommendations on Limits for Exposure to Ionizing Radiations*, NCRP, Bethesda, MD, 1987.

Performance and responsibility guidelines for NMT, SNM Technologists Section, *J. Nucl. Med.*, 44, 222, 2003.

Saha, G.B., *Physics and Radiobiology of Nuclear Medicine*, Springer–Verlag, New York, 1993.

Saha, G.B., *Basics of PET Imaging*, Springer, New York, 2005.

Sandler, M.P., Coleman, R.E., Patton, J.A., Wackers, F.J., and Gottschalk, A., Editors, *Diagnostic Nuclear Medicine*, Lippincott Williams, & Wilkins, Philadelphia, 2003.

Shackett, P., *Nuclear Medicine Technology — Procedures and Quick Reference*, Lippincott Williams & Wilkins, Philadelphia, 2000.

Silverstein, E.B., Radionuclides and radiopharmaceuticals for 2005, *J. Nucl. Med.*, 46, 13N, 2005.

Steves, A.M., *Review of Nuclear Medicine Technology*, 2d ed., Society of Nuclear Medicine, Reston, VA, 1996.

Technetium Tc-99m Generator for Diagnostic Use, package insert, Bristol–Myers Squibb, N. Billerica, 2003.

Turner, J.E., Editor, *Atoms, Radiation, and Radiation Protection*, 2d ed., John Willey & Sons, Inc., New York, 1995.

Wagner, H.N., Administration guidelines for radioimmunotherapy of non-Hodgkins lymphoma with ^{90}Y-labeled anti-CD20 MoAb, *J. Nucl. Med.*, 43, 267, 2002.

6 Safe Handling of Radioactivity

I. RATIONALE

The NM department is a radiation-clean, radiation-safe environment in which patients are cared for during the diagnostic and therapeutic tests needed to alleviate their illnesses. Radiation workers (radiopharmacists, NMTs, and nuclear physicians) must pay close attention to every step of each procedure to ensure the safety of the patients, the staff, and the visitors. According to the ALARA policy, all exposures must be minimized and all unnecessary exposures prevented.

Exposure to radiation occurs in just about every task performed in the NM department:

1. Preparation and QA of radiopharmaceuticals
2. Diagnostic imaging procedures, including PET/CT
3. QA testing of gamma cameras, nuclide generators, dose calibrators, and survey meters
4. Radionuclide therapy procedures

This chapter deals with the basic principles and methods used by radiation workers to minimize their external and internal exposures, the laboratory rules they must follow, and the recognition of radiation hazards in their working environment.

II. MINIMIZING EXTERNAL EXPOSURES

A. Principles

1. Quantity of Radioactivity Used

The quantity of radioactivity used in each procedure is the minimum amount that will produce a high-quality result. Examples are (a) the mCi (MBq) quantities used in imaging procedures which show valuable diagnostic information about the patient's illness and (b) the nCi (Bq) quantities used in a radiochemical purity test of a RP by thin-layer chromatography (TLC).

Figure 6.1 shows that the exposure rate is directly and linearly related to the quantity of the radioactivity used. Doubling the radioactivity doubles the exposure rate; reducing the amount of radioactivity used reduces the exposure rate proportionally. Thus, if the

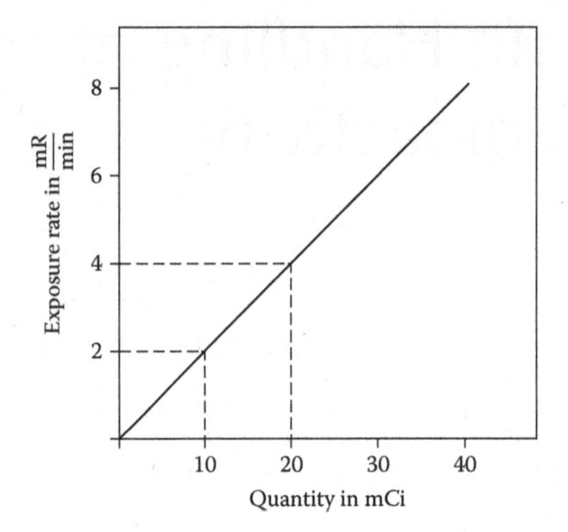

FIGURE 6.1 Exposure rate is linearly related to the quantity of radioactivity used. Doubling the quantity doubles the exposure rate.

hands of a technologist are exposed to 2 mR/min during the loading of a syringe with 10 mCi (370 MBq) of a radioactive solution, loading it with 20 mCi (740 MBq) would expose the hands to a rate of 4 mR/min.

2. Time of Exposure

Practice makes perfect. Practice reduces the time needed to prepare RPs, to dispense individual dosages, and to inject RPs. To minimize exposure, the time of exposure must be minimized. Figure 6.2 shows that total exposure is directly and linearly

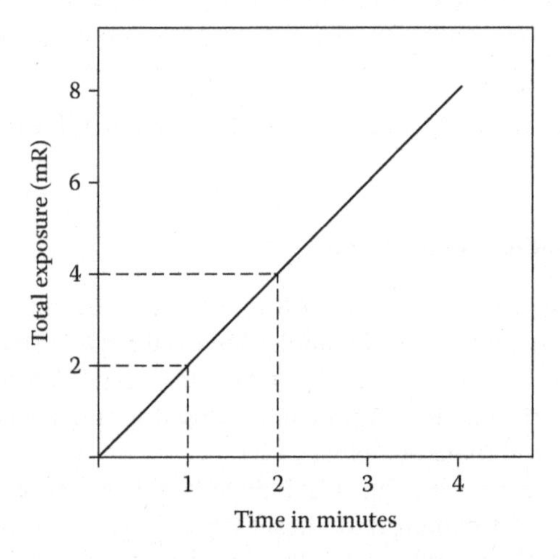

FIGURE 6.2 Total exposure is linearly related to exposure time. Doubling the time doubles the total exposure.

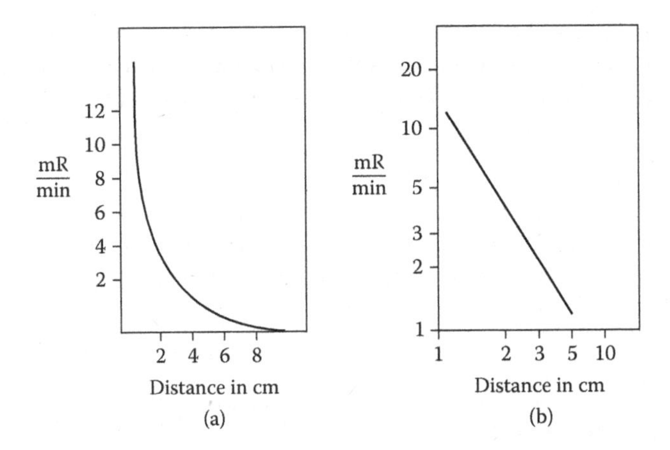

FIGURE 6.3 Exposure rate decreases inversely with the square of the distance: (a) linear graph, (b) logarithmic graph.

related to time. Doubling the time it takes to perform a task doubles the total exposure. Total exposure is equal to the product of exposure rate and time:

$$\text{Total Exposure (total mR)} = \text{Exposure Rate (mR/min)} \times \text{Time (min)} \quad (6.1)$$

In the same fashion, total dose in μSv is equal to dose rate in μSv/min × time in minutes. Thus, improving the skill to load syringes with radioactive solutions would reduce the time needed to perform such task and, therefore, reduce exposure.

3. Effect of Distance

When reading a book, moving closer to the light source improves the illumination, because more light photons reach the book. When working with radioactivity, moving closer to the source means higher exposure too; moving away means lower exposure. For point sources, exposure rate is inversely related to the square of the distance. This fact is known as the *inverse square law.* Figure 6.3(a) shows that the curve is a hyperbola, a power function of distance, which can be linearized (converted into a straight line) by plotting the data on logarithmic graph paper (Figure 6.3(b).

The same principle applies to any phenomenon in which particles, rays, or galaxies move from a center of emission into space. Examples are the light emission from a light bulb, camera flash, the explosion of a grenade, an atomic bomb shock wave, the galaxies moving away from each other after the Big Bang, and, of course, the rays coming from a radioactive vial. The reason is that, if you double the radius of a sphere, the surface area quadruples, and, therefore, the *flux*, which is the number of rays per unit of surface area, decreases to one-fourth. For those who may wish to verify this statement, the formula of the surface of a sphere is

$$S = 4\pi r^2 \quad (6.2)$$

Similarly, tripling the distance reduces the exposure or dose rate to one-ninth, etc., and, by the same token, halving the distance increases the exposure rate by a factor of four. A practical formula is

$$I_1 \times D_1^2 = I_2 \times D_2^2 \tag{6.3}$$

where I_1 = given intensity or exposure rate, I_2 = given intensity or asked exposure rate, D_1 = given distance, and D_2 = given or asked distance.

Sample Problems

(a) The dose rate at 10 cm from a ^{99m}Tc generator is 18 μSv/h. What would the dose rate be at 12 in.?
Solution: First, we must convert inches to cm: 12 in. × 2.54 cm/in. = 30.48 cm. Now we can apply Equation 6.3 to obtain 1.94 μSv/h (answer).

(b) The exposure rate at 25 cm from a radioactive source is 45 mR/h (450 μSv/h). At what distance will the exposure rate drop to 5 mR/h (50 μSv/h)?
Solution: Just a glance at the problem would reveal that 5 is 1/9 of 45; therefore, tripling the distance would reduce the exposure rate to 5 mR/h (50 μSv/h). However, using Equation 6.3 would prove it mathematically:

$$45 \times 25^2 = 5 \times D_2^2$$

$$D_2 = 75 \text{ cm (answer)}$$

Comment: Although a radioactive patient is by no means a point source, the inverse square law can be used to obtain an acceptable estimate of the exposure rate at some distance from a high-uptake organ even before injecting the patient. The same is true for estimating the exposure or dose rate from a vial containing any radioactive pharmaceutical. To do this, we need the *specific gamma constant*, which gives the exposure rate per mCi or per GBq of each radionuclide (see Table 2.4 and Appendix C). Awareness of the effect of distance is essential to minimizing external exposures.

4. Effect of Shielding

The use of shielding is one of the most practical ways of reducing exposures in the NM department. This is especially true in the hot lab, where relatively large amounts of radioactivity are handled daily.

Principle: For collimated (narrow) beams of x- or gamma rays, the transmitted intensity decreases exponentially with linear increases of shield thickness. Figure 6.4 shows a collimated beam of gamma rays, a scintillation detector, and a shield between the two. The radiation being measured by the detector is the attenuated

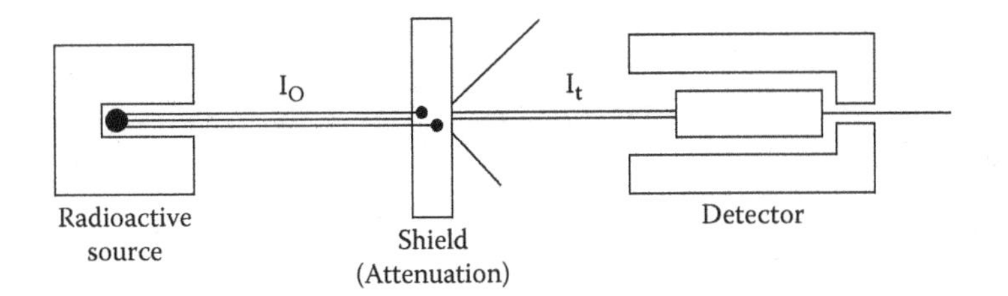

FIGURE 6.4 For collimated (narrow) beams of gamma rays, the transmitted intensity decreases exponentially with linear increases of shield thickness. Attenuation is the result of absorption and deflection of gamma rays within the shield.

beam. Attenuation is the result of absorption of gamma rays in the shield by photoelectric effect and the deflection of gamma rays in the shield by Compton effect. And, the thicker the shield, the greater is the degree of attenuation. The equation that describes this phenomenon is the following:

$$I_t = I_0 e^{-\mu x} \tag{6.4}$$

where I_t = transmitted intensity, I_0 = original intensity, e = base of the natural logarithms (1.71828...), μ = attenuation coefficient, and x = shield thickness.

When x is measured in linear units (cm or in.), the attenuation coefficient μ becomes the *linear attenuation coefficient* μ_L, which is defined as the fractional attenuation per unit of linear thickness. When x is expressed as density thickness units (g/cm^2), μ becomes the *mass attenuation coefficient* μ_M, defined as the fractional attenuation per unit of density thickness.

Most medical personnel prefer the linear approach, which is the one used in this book. Physicists prefer the density thickness approach. Regardless of the approach, however, the attenuation coefficient is an expression of the quality of the shielding material as an attenuator of gamma or x-rays. Further, the two expressions are related by the following equation:

$$\mu_L = \mu_M \times \rho \tag{6.5}$$

where ρ = density of material in g/cm^3.

A practical way to deal with shielding problems is the application of the half-value layer (HVL), which is defined as the thickness that reduces the intensity of a gamma or x-ray beam to one-half of its original value. Figure 6.5(a) shows that the transmitted intensity decreases exponentially with linear increases of shield thickness. Figure 6.5(b) shows that the exponential curve is linearized by plotting the data on semilogarithmic graph paper. The figure shows the attenuation of a narrow beam of ^{137}Cs gamma rays by lead. Also shown is the HVL of 0.61 cm of lead. Mathematically, it can be shown that HVL = ln 2/μ_L and that μ_L = ln 2/HVL, which are extremely useful formulas when calculating thicknesses of materials to be used as shields in NM or "filters" in radiology.

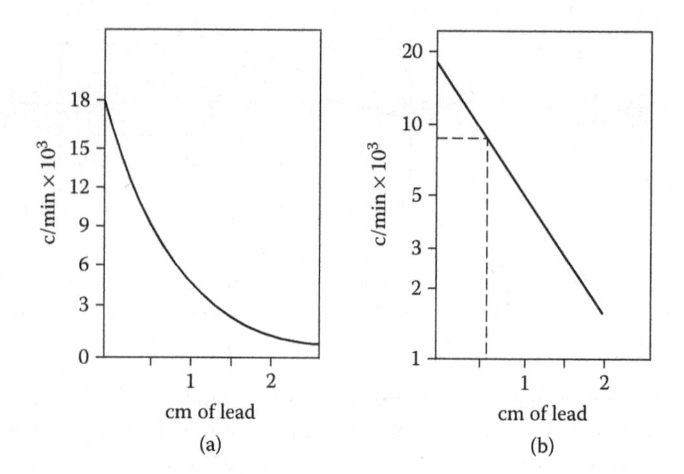

FIGURE 6.5 Count rate or exposure rate decreases exponentially with linear increases of shield thickness: (a) linear graph, (b) semilogarithmic graph.

Sample Problems

(a) The dose rate on the surface of a ^{99m}Tc generator is 350 μSv/h. What would the exposure rate be if the generator were placed just behind a lead shield 1/2-in. thick?
Solution: First, we are dealing with the parent of ^{99m}Tc: ^{99}Mo, whose most important gamma rays have energies of 740 and 780 keV. The HVL is 0.7 cm of lead. Second, the thickness of the shield (0.5 in.) must be converted to centimeters of lead: 0.5 in. × 2.54 cm/in. = 1.27 cm. Third, we must apply the attenuation equation as follows:

$$I_t = 350e^{-0.693 \times 1.27/0.7}$$

$$I_t = 350 \times 0.2843 = 99.5 \ \mu\text{Sv/h (answer)}$$

where 0.693 = ln 2 and 0.2843 = attenuation factor, "the fraction … passing through."

(b) In a similar situation to that of the previous case, what would the thickness of a lead shield be to reduce an exposure rate from 350 to 20 μSv/h?
Solution: By substituting in the attenuation equation,

$$20 = 350e^{-0.693x/0.7}$$

In this case, the unknown is x, the thickness of the shield, which is part of the exponent. Formal procedure calls for transfer of 350 to the left, taking the reciprocal of the second member of the equation (this step removes the negative sign). Then, by flipping both fractions, applying

TABLE 6.1
Estimation of Attenuation Factors

Number of HVLs	Attenuation Factor
1	0.5
2	0.25
3	0.125
4	0.0625
5	0.03125
6	0.015625
7	0.0078125
8	0.00390625
3.3	0.10 (10%)
6.6	0.01 (1%)
9.9	0.001 (0.1%)

natural logs on both sides, and solving for x, the answer is x = 2.89 cm of lead.

Table 6.1 shows that the definition of HVL allows us to make reasonable estimates to questions of shielding before we apply the shielding equation. Table 6.2 gives the HVLs of the most widely used medical radionuclides. Figure 6.6 shows

TABLE 6.2
Half-Value Layers of Medical Radionuclides

Symbol	Main (Average) Energies (keV)	HVL (mm of Pb)
^{125}I	27–32 (30)	0.2
^{201}Tl	69–83 (76)	0.2
^{133}Xe	81	0.2
^{57}Co	123	0.2
^{99m}Tc	140	0.25
^{123}I	159	0.4
^{67}Ga	93, 184, 296, 388 (174)	0.66
^{111}In	173, 247 (210)	0.72
^{51}Cr	320	1.7
^{131}I	364	2.2
^{11}C	511	4.0
^{15}O	511	4.0
^{68}Ga	511	4.0
^{18}F	511	4.1
^{137}Cs	662	6.1
^{82}Rb	511, 780 (544)	7.0
^{99}Mo	740, 780 (636)	7.0
^{60}Co	1,110; 1,330 (1.25)	12.0

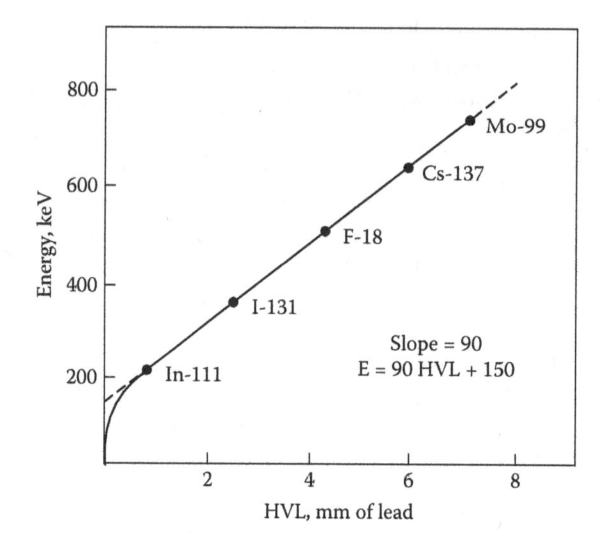

FIGURE 6.6 Between 200 and 800 keV, there is a linear relationship between gamma energy and HVLs of lead.

that, between 200 and 800 keV, HVLs are linear with energies. The slope of that portion of the curve is 90 keV/mm of lead and the y-intercept is 150 keV. In that range, the following equation could be used to calculate HVLs or, given the HVL, the corresponding energy:

$$E = 90\ \text{HVL} + 150 \tag{6.6}$$

III. PREVENTING INTERNAL CONTAMINATION

Internal contamination is possible, but it is not probable in a radiation safety-conscious department. If it occurs, the most likely routes of entry are by ingestion, inhalation, percutaneous absorption, or by accidental injection.

A. Ingestion

Compliance with one basic laboratory rule of safety will prevent accidental ingestion of radioactivity: there should be no eating, drinking, or using cosmetics in the working areas of the NM department. To this, we may add: there should be no gum chewing or use of mints or lozenges. All these activities should be done in the staff lounge. There is no need to mention smoking, which is not permitted anywhere in the hospital. By the same token, no laboratory coats, gloves, or radioactivity of any kind should be brought into the lounge room, the waiting room, and the clerical offices.

B. Inhalation

Some gaseous radioactivities, such as ^{133}Xe, ^{127}Xe, or ^{81m}Kr, and some volatile radioactivities, such as ^{131}I or ^{125}I, could be released accidentally in some working areas. But there are ways to prevent such releases, as well as to control them if they should occur. There are also ways to make sure that releases do not occur inadvertently. The latter calls for special monitoring techniques. All these methods are aimed at ensuring that inhalation of radioactivities does not occur. Following are some of those preventive measures:

1. Administration of ^{133}Xe, ^{127}Xe, or ^{81m}Kr gases during pulmonary ventilation studies is normally done using a sealed dispensing system. Technologists instruct the patient about what is to be done and even rehearse the procedure before administration. This ensures a successful study. The room has an air extractor, which directs the flow of air from the front to the back and away from the staff should an accidental release occur. The room door is closed to prevent the flow of gas into the hall. When the study is completed, the gas is returned to a shielded container, where it is trapped in charcoal canisters to remain in storage until decay is complete.
2. Of special concern are therapeutic solutions of ^{131}I and ^{125}I. The reason is that these radionuclides can become airborne if kept in neutral or acid solutions. Volatilization can be prevented if such solutions are kept in alkaline pH. This is not always possible when they are to be administered to patients. Thus, proper handling of such solutions is imperative. First, all preparations are to be done in a properly operating fume hood or glove box. Second, the exhaust must be equipped with sodium hydroxide solution traps to catch any volatile radioiodine. Third, any liquid waste must be dumped in a container with some strong NaOH solution and kept covered. This container must be placed behind lead shielding on the back of the hood. Patients and their nurses must receive written instructions regarding radiation safety and emergencies.

C. Percutaneous Absorption

1. Percutaneous absorption is the entry of radioactivity through the pores of the skin. Of special concern are tritium (^{3}H) and ^{14}C-compounds being used in certain medical research laboratories. In NM departments, all liquid radioactivities are important, but especially important are therapeutic solutions of ^{131}I, ^{125}I, ^{89}Sr, ^{90}Y, ^{153}Sm, and ^{32}P. See also Table 1.4 for the physical properties of negatron emitters and Table 6.3 for their therapeutic applications. They are to be handled with special attention to safety. The key is to prevent contact with the skin. Long-sleeved laboratory coats, gloves, masking tapes around the wrists to seal the gap between the gloves and the lab coat sleeves, transparent plastic shields in front of the face, and lead–glass glasses or goggles are recommended when handling these nuclides in liquid form. With these precautionary measures, should an accidental spill occur, contact with the skin does not happen. Some laboratories use a glove box or a fume hood to prepare therapeutic doses of beta emitters.

TABLE 6.3
Radionuclide Therapy

Illness	Radiopharmaceutical
B-cell lymphomas, LB leukemia	^{90}Y-ibritumomab, ^{90}Y-rituximab
GI, breast, ovarian, lung cancers	^{125}I-B72.3 (murine MAb)
Hepatocellular carcinoma	^{90}Y-microspheres
Hyperthyroidism, thyroid cancer	^{131}I-sodium iodide
Intracavitary malignancies	^{32}P-chromic phosphate suspension
Neuroendocrine tumors	^{90}Y-pentetreotide
Non-Hodgkins lymphoma	^{90}Y-epratuzomab, ^{131}I-tositumomab
Ovarian cancer	^{32}P-colloid, ^{90}Y-colloid, ^{186}Re-HEDP
Palliation of pain in bone metastases	^{89}Sr-chloride, ^{32}P-phosphate, ^{153}Sm-EDTMP
Polycythemia vera, leukemia	^{32}P-sodium phosphate

2. PET imaging agents are usually prepared in unit dosages and require a minimum of handling at the time of injection. However, if received in multiple dosage vials, the dispensation of individual dosages, transportation to the imaging room, and injection require proper and heavy shielding: L-block shields, with lead-glass windows 4-in. thick, a shielded enclosure for handling the vial, lead–glass goggles, lead boxes for transporting the individual shielded syringes, etc. Remember that the HVL for 511 keV annihilation radiation photons is 4.1 mm of lead and 2.8 mm of tungsten. Specially designed tungsten syringe shields are recommended.
3. If contamination of the skin does occur accidentally, the contaminated clothing must be removed immediately, and decontamination of the skin with soap and water must follow. This is followed by proper monitoring to ensure successful decontamination. Some cases may require special decontamination procedures (see reference by Schleien, Chapter 11, pages 11–92).

D. Accidental Injection

To prevent accidental needle stings, the staff must develop and maintain their skills in handling needles and syringes. The concern is not limited to possible contamination with radioactivities but also with biohazards such as the hepatitis B virus and the human immunodeficiency virus (HIV).

Each hospital or clinic has a policy on proper handling of used needles on disposable syringes so as to prevent accidental stings. Those policies must be heeded.

IV. LABORATORY RULES

1. No person shall handle radioactive materials without wearing a film badge or a pocket dosimeter.
2. Personal belongings should not be brought to the laboratory.

3. Eating, drinking, or using cosmetics in the laboratory is forbidden.
4. Lab coats and gloves must be worn when handling radioactivity and/or biological fluids.
5. All laboratory benches and trays must be covered with absorbent paper with impermeable backing.
6. Lab coats and disposable gloves must not be brought to nonrestricted areas. They are considered contaminated.
7. Monitoring of working areas must be done at the license-prescribed intervals.
8. Before leaving the laboratory, monitoring of hands and clothing is required.
9. All radioactive substances and all dosages must be correctly labeled.
10. Solid and liquid wastes must be disposed as prescribed by the license.
11. Appropriate radiation warning signs must be placed as prescribed by the NRC.
12. Fume hood fans must always be on unless there is a reason for turning them off. In such cases, the front glass must be closed.
13. When preparing dosages, proper aseptic techniques must be applied.
14. Good housekeeping of the laboratory is imperative.

V. RADIATION HAZARDS

A. Alpha Emitters

Alpha emitters have no diagnostic applications in NM. Radium-226 needles were used in therapy some years ago and they may still be in storage in some facilities. They have platinum capsules 0.5-mm thick that stop all particle radiations emitted by ^{226}Ra and its descendants. Their therapeutic effect is due to very high-intensity gamma and x-ray emissions. Rupture of the capsule can result in release of radioactivities, including ^{222}Rn, the daughter of ^{226}Ra, and also an alpha emitter. ^{222}Rn is a gas that can enter the body by inhalation. Alpha particles are high-LET radiations. Their radiation weighting factor is 20. Their range in air is about 3 to 4 cm and in soft tissue about 20 μm. Figure 6.7 is a microscopic autoradiograph in which a source of ^{210}Po appears on the intestinal mucosa of a laboratory animal. The alpha particle tracks are clearly shown in the photographic emulsion that coats the tissue section. Externally, alpha particles cannot cross the dead layer of the skin, which is about 70-μm thick. Internally, however, they would kill any cell they hit in the bronchial mucosa, in the lungs' alveoli, in the gastrointestinal lining, etc.

In accordance with NRC regulations, all alpha sources greater than 10 μCi must be leak-tested at 6-month intervals, and records must be kept. For sealed sources emitting beta radiation, leak-testing is required for activities greater than 100 μCi. A test is positive when it can be shown that it exceeds 0.005 μCi (185 Bq) of removable radioactivity. For ^{222}Rn, leakage greater than 1 nCi/24 h (37 Bq/24 h) is considered positive. Monitoring of alpha radiation contamination, as well as leak testing, is done by wipe or swab techniques. Quantification is achieved using suitable standards.

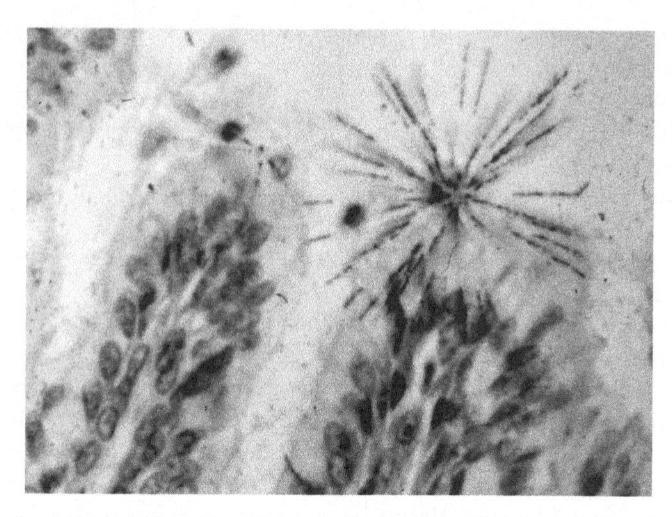

FIGURE 6.7 Microscopic autoradiograph of the intestine of a mouse. In soft tissues, Po-210 alpha particles have a range about equal to the length of a cylindrical cell, or approximately 20 μm.

B. Negatron Emitters

1. In diagnostic procedures, negatrons are incidental to the measurement of gamma radiation. Gamma rays, and in some cases x-rays, are the ones that make up the images. The most important diagnostic negatron-gamma emitters are ^{131}I and ^{133}Xe. ^{131}I is used in the thyroid uptake test, but only in microcurie quantities because of its negatron emissions (1.3 rad or 13 mGy to the gland per microcurie). ^{133}Xe is used in lung ventilation studies. A typical adult dose is 10 mCi (370 MBq), but only because its biological half-life is about 20 s.
2. On the other hand, in radionuclide therapy, negatrons deliver the needed radiation dose to stop the progress of the illness and possibly cure the patient. A high radiation dose is needed to treat the malignant tissues. For example, ^{131}I is used in doses of 10 to 29 mCi (370 to 1,073 MBq) to treat hyperthyroidism, and in doses of 30 to 300 mCi (1.11 to 11.1 GBq) to treat thyroid cancer. In the case of ^{125}I, 93% of the 35-keV gamma rays emitted undergo internal conversion, which results in the emission of monoenergetic conversion electrons. In effect then, ^{125}I behaves like a negatron emitter. Consequently, its use is reserved to in vitro radioassays and to therapy.
3. Other negatron emitters: ^{32}P, which is a pure negatron emitter, is used to treat polycythemia vera with phosphate solutions and intracavitary malignancies with colloidal phosphate suspensions; ^{90}Sr and its daughter ^{90}Y are pure negatron emitters. They are used in topical therapy of ocular tumors. In addition, ^{90}Y, bound to antibodies through a chelating agent, is used to treat non-Hodgkins lymphoma (NHL). Negatrons have a radi-

ation weighting factor of 1, meaning that they produce less than 100 ion pairs/μm in soft tissue. Table 1.4 gives the main properties of some negatron emitters, and Table 6.3 gives their therapeutic applications.

4. Monitoring for possible contamination with negatron emitters depends on the energy and the quantity of the spill. For low-level energy or quantities, the wipe technique must be used. For high-energy negatrons, a portable survey meter may be sufficient. Hazards depend on the chemical form, energy, and quantity of radioactivity. In soft tissues, negatrons can penetrate from a few microns to 12 mm depending on the energy. Recommended shielding materials are those of low atomic number, such as glass, plastic, or aluminum, which minimize the production of bremsstrahlung (braking radiation).
5. The hazard of beta radiation can be estimated with the following equation:

$$D_\beta = 760\ A \tag{6.7}$$

where D_β = dose rate in μSv/h at 10 cm from a point source and A = activity in MBq.

Sample Problem

What is the dose rate at 25 cm from a vial containing 400 MBq of ^{32}P-phosphate solution?

Solution:

a. $D_\beta = 760 \times 400 = 304{,}000$ μSv/h = 304 mSv/h at 10 cm.
b. At 25 cm (inverse square law) = 48.6 mSv/h (answer).
c. Recommendation: Use a plastic shield.

C. Positron Emitters

Table 1.5 lists the most important positron emitters used in NM. Among them, ^{18}F in the form of fluorodeoxyglucose (FDG) is the most widely used in positron emission tomography (PET) applications. This is due to its very special properties: a half-life of 110 min, its ability to substitute for hydrogen in organic molecules, E_{max} of 635 keV, range in tissue of 2.4 mm, LET of 0.27 keV/μm. Regional medical cyclotrons produce ^{18}F-FDG, which is synthesized by radiochemical synthesizers (robotic devices) and then distributed to hospitals and clinics within a radius of a 2-h flight. The interest in FDG rests on the fact that it is an excellent metabolic radiotracer for the brain, the myocardium, and for tumors. In addition, it is well quantified by PET. Many gamma cameras have dual capability: single-photon emission tomography (SPECT) and PET. More recently, the merging of PET scanners and computerized tomography (CT) has revolutionized the practice of NM. Please see a description in Chapter 4. Other positron emitters, such as ^{11}C, ^{13}N, and ^{15}O, remain mostly as research tools, with very limited use in routine clinical practice because of their very short half-lives. ^{68}Ga and ^{82}Rb are obtained from nuclide generators, but they have serious limitations. For example, ^{68}Ga requires 2 to 4 d to complete a diagnostic study, and its half-life is only 68 min. ^{82}Rb has a half-life of only 75 s.

In addition to bremsstrahlung, positrons produce annihilation radiation: two 511 keV photons. Thus, positron sources require heavy shielding. The HVL of lead for 511 keV photons is 16 times that of ^{99m}Tc, or about 4.1 mm of lead. Monitoring of ^{18}F can be done similarly to any gamma emitter. Hazards of positron emitters are similar to those of negatron emitters.

D. Gamma Emitters

Table 6.2 shows some gamma emitters, their main gamma or x-ray emissions, and their HVLs.

Most of them are electron capture–gamma emitting radionuclides. ^{99m}Tc is an isomeric transition-gamma emitting radionuclide. Some are negatron–gamma emitters. Some are positron emitters and annihilation radiation radionuclides. Some have abundant daughters' x-ray emissions. In all cases, photon emissions are low-LET radiations and have a radiation weighting factor of 1.

Photons of energies less than 100 keV are largely absorbed in bone. Photons of energies less than 50 keV are significantly absorbed in soft tissue. For example, the half-value-layer of soft tissue for ^{99m}Tc gamma rays is 4.5 cm. The same for ^{201}Tl is 3.8 cm. Monitoring for gamma emitter contamination depends on the energy of the gamma emissions and on the quantity of the radioactivity. For low quantities and low energies, the wipe technique is used. Wipes are measured with a well-type gamma counter connected to a single- or multichannel analyzer and a printer. Some wipe-counters are specially designed for ^{99m}Tc gamma emissions (Figure 7.1). The software may allow calculations and reporting of results automatically. For high levels or high energies, a gamma survey meter may be used.

E. Neutrons

Although neutrons are not used in diagnostic NM, they are considered a therapeutic modality for the not-too-distant future. Neutrons can penetrate deeply in the body and cause spallation of carbon and oxygen nuclei into three and four alpha particles, respectively, right inside the tumor. Neutrons do not ionize atoms and molecules directly, but they do so by secondary means: they set protons into motion, and these are highly ionizing.

To shield against neutrons, low-atomic-number materials are necessary. This is due to the fact that neutrons transfer a large fraction of their kinetic energy to the small nuclei with which they collide. Thus, they can be "stopped" with a smaller number of collisions if the material contains low-Z elements. Examples of good attenuators of neutrons are paraffin and water, which are rich in hydrogen; graphite, which is carbon; and polyethylene, which is rich in both hydrogen and carbon.

Neutron hazards: If a radiation worker is accidentally exposed to a shower of neutrons, several types of reactions can occur in the body:

1. Neutron capture-gamma reaction with hydrogen: H(n, γ)D. The product deuterium (D) is a heavy, nonradioactive isotope of hydrogen (H-2).

2. Activation of ^{23}Na to ^{24}Na, also by neutron capture, but the product is a negatron–gamma emitter, which decays with a 15-h half-life.
3. Production of ^{14}C by a neutron-proton reaction with nitrogen: $^{14}N(n, p)^{14}C$. Carbon-14 is a pure negatron emitter with a half-life of 5,730 y. Thus, depending on the dose, internal irradiation can be severe.

The best monitors for neutrons are proportional counters filled with boron fluoride gas, which is very efficient at detecting thermal neutrons. For fast neutrons, the detector may be surrounded with polyethylene or another neutron attenuator. The neutron–boron interaction is as follows:

$$^{10}B(n, \alpha)^{7}Li$$

VI. RADIONUCLIDE THERAPY

Radionuclide therapy involves the use of relatively large quantities of beta-emitters with half-lives measured in weeks. Special handling procedures are required. Patient excretions may contain large amounts of radioactivity during the first 24 to 72 h after dosing. Table 6.3 gives some of the most common therapeutic procedures and the therapeutic agents used.

Perhaps the most frequent procedure is the use of ^{131}I therapy for hyperthyroidism and thyroid cancer. That procedure is used here to describe the radiation-safety-handling techniques.

A. Radioiodine Therapy

Iodine-131 is used in three procedures, which differ in nature as well as in the level of radioactivity given to the patient. The NM physician and the RSO supervise the procedures.

1. Imaging of Metastases

Imaging is performed approximately six months after surgery. The dose range is about 1 to 5 mCi (37 to 185 MBq) of sodium iodide as a capsule or drinking solution. A special formulation of the solution minimizes volatilization of ^{131}I.

2. Hyperthyroidism

a. Grave's disease: 5 to 10 mCi (185 to 370 MBq) dosage
b. Plummer's disease: 10 to 29 mCi (370 to 1073 MBq) dosage

3. Thyroid Ablation

Ablation usually follows surgery. The range of doses is 100 to 300 mCi (3.7 to 11.1 GBq). Bioassay testing of the staff involved in dosing and caring for the patient is required. Detailed documentation of every step of the procedure is required.

B. Thyroid Ablation

Patient isolation is required. Because ^{131}I will appear in the urine, saliva, perspiration, tears, and other body fluids, some precautions are taken:

1. In the patient's isolation room, floors and walls are covered with absorbent paper with impermeable backing and secured with masking tape.
2. Door knobs, the telephone, the nurse-calling device, the TV remote control, and other objects are covered with transparent plastic bags.
3. Two radioactive waste containers, labeled with radiation warning signs, are placed near the bed and near the entrance.
4. The bed mattress and the pillows are covered with plastic and then with the linens. Plenty of clean linens are placed in a closet for quick changes.
5. A cooler containing water and soft drinks is placed in the room for the patient's use. The patient is encouraged to drink plenty of fluids and to void frequently.
6. A line is marked on the floor 3 m from the bed. Visitors are instructed not to cross the line.
7. A radiation warning sign is placed on the door, indicating the amount of radioactivity used and the nurse attending times, based on monitorings of the patient. Other radiation warning signs are placed on the bed, the patient's chart, and the patient's wrist.
8. Hospital staff are instructed not to perform their housekeeping duties in that room during the stay of the patient.
9. On a table outside the room, a GM survey meter or an ion chamber instrument is set to perform frequent monitorings. Exposure rate on the outside walls or adjacent rooms should not exceed 2 mR/h (20 μSv/h).
10. A practical way of determining the amount of activity remaining in the patient is to take a measurement of the exposure rate at 3 meters from the patient immediately after the administration of the dosage. That measurement represents the 100% reading. Similar readings at 24 h, 48 h, 72 h, etc., will then represent the fraction or percentage remaining at those times.

Patient care includes:

a. The nurse assigned to the patient is considered a radiation worker. He or she must wear a film or TLD badge or a pocket dosimeter and must be instructed on how to read the pocket dosimeter and to keep records.
b. Attending times are determined by the RSO and posted on the room door. For example, for a patient who receives a 100-mCi (3.7 GBq) dosage of ^{131}I, the total times in which a nurse would receive 100 mrem (1 mSv) are 1.5 h at 2 ft and 15 h at 6 ft. The total time is divided by 10 d. That would result in 9 min/d at 2 ft and 90 min/d at 6 ft. The nurse wears disposable gloves and shoe covers every time he or she enters the room. Those items are removed upon leaving the room and disposed in the radioactive waste container by the door.

c. The patient receives instructions verbally and in writing about being confined to the room for the duration of the therapy (5 to 7 d) and about the use of food trays, food waste, use of the facilities, etc. He or she is also given the telephone numbers to call in case of emergencies.
d. No pregnant nurses, NMTs, or visitors are allowed. No visitors under age 18 are allowed. No visitors are allowed during the first 24 h.

C. Release of Patients

1. A patient may be released when the dose to any other individual close to the patient will not exceed 500 mrem (5 mSv). If the dose is likely to exceed 100 mrem (1 mSv), the medical institution must provide the patient with written instructions on actions to maintain doses to others ALARA. If there are children or pregnant women at home, the release of the patient may be delayed.
2. If, for other reasons, the patient needs to be hospitalized, he or she can be transferred to a semi-private room.

D. Room Decontamination

1. NMTs doing the decontamination wear gloves and shoe covers. They remove paper coverings and place them in plastic bags. They monitor the room and every object in it. Food trays, eating utensils, and other objects are placed in plastic bags. All linens are placed in plastic bags. Plastic bags that read more than 5 mR/h (50 μSv/h) are either stored to decay or disposed as radioactive waste.
2. The bathroom is scrubbed clean. Monitoring should result in less than 5 mR/h (50 μSv/h). When monitoring shows that the room is clean, the hospital staff is informed so that housekeeping can be restored, and admitting is informed that the room is available.

VII. OTHER RADIONUCLIDE THERAPIES

A. Phosphorus-32

1. Phosphorus-32 is used in the form of ^{32}P-phosphate, to treat polycythemia vera and to palliate pain of bone metastases from malignant illnesses. Usual dosages are 5 to 10 mCi (185 to 370 MBq). The vial and the syringe containing the RP must use special shields made of lead lined with plastic, usually acrylic. The plastic is to stop most of the beta particles and to minimize bremsstrahlung radiation. The lead is to attenuate the latter. Depending on the condition of the patient, he or she may be hospitalized. Because ^{32}P is a pure beta emitter, nurses do not have to wear film or TLD badges. Patient care, prevention of decontamination, and decontamination procedures are similar to those described for radioiodine.

2. In the form of colloidal suspension, ^{32}P is used to treat intracavitary malignancies. The RP is usually administered by instillation directly into the affected cavity (pleural or peritoneal) in dosages of 5 to 20 mCi (185 to 740 MBq). Patients may be hospitalized. Contamination of linens is possible if there is leakage of radioactivity from the instillation site. Disposable linens are recommended. Attendants must wear gloves.

B. Strontium-89 Chloride and ^{153}Sm-EDTMP

These two agents are used to alleviate pain of bone metastases from malignant disease. Safety precautions are similar to those of ^{32}P. EDTMP stands for ethylene diamine tetramethylene phosphonic acid. ^{153}Sm is a beta emitter with a significant gamma component, and, therefore, handling requires special shielding devices. To avoid harm at the site of injection due to infiltration, administration should be done through an intravenous line. Disposable linens are recommended.

C. Yttrium-90

Yttrium-90 is a high-energy negatron emitter that decays with a half-life of 64 h. Some examples of its applications follow.

a. Bound to biocompatible microspheres, it can be injected into the hepatic artery to treat liver metastatic tumors from colorectal cancer.
b. Bound to rituximab, a humanized monoclonal (chimeric) antibody, it is used in the treatment of non-Hodgkins lymphoma and acute lymphoblastic leukemias. In this case, ^{90}Y is bound to the antibody through a chelating agent. Rituximab targets CD20, a specific surface antigen on normal and malignant B-lymphocytes.
c. Another example is ^{90}Y-Ibritumomab tiuxetan, a murine radioimmuno-conjugate that binds the CD20 surface antigen on B-cells and, therefore, is indicated for the same malignancies as rituximab.

D. Iodine-125

Iodine-125, bound to B72.3, a murine monoclonal antibody that targets TAG-72, a glycoprotein antigen, is used to treat colon, esophageal, gastric, breast, pancreatic, ovarian cancer, and non-small-cell lung carcinomas.

E. Iodine-131

Iodine-131 bound to tositumomab, a murine monoclonal antibody, that targets CD20, is used to treat non-Hodgkins lymphoma.

PROBLEMS

1. The dose rate at 25 cm from a radioactive source is 340 μSv/h. At what distance will the rate drop to 50 μSv/h?
2. The dose rate at the desk of a laboratory supervisor was found to be 30 μSv/h. The reason is that there was a ^{99m}Tc generator in the next room without shielding toward the office. If the HVL of ^{99}Mo gamma rays is 0.7 cm of lead, what thickness of lead would reduce the dose rate to 1 μSv/h in accordance with the ALARA policy?
3. Using a pair of tongs, a technologist holds and swirls a multidosage vial behind a lead-glass shield for 2 min. The hand dosimeter later reads 180 μSv. What would the hand dose be if the swirling time were reduced to one minute?
4. The dose rate on the surface of a ^{99m}Tc generator is 360 μSv/h. What thickness of lead would have to be added to reduce the rate to 20 μSv/h?
5. The linear attenuation coefficient of soft tissue for the 27-keV x-rays of ^{125}I is 0.45 cm^{-1}. What fraction of those x-rays will penetrate 2.5 cm of soft tissue?
6. The HVL of lead for ^{99m}Tc gamma rays is 0.025 cm. What fraction of those gamma rays will pass through a lead apron 1-mm thick?
7. A ^{99m}Tc generator arrives Monday morning. A quick survey of the package results in an exposure rate of 750 μSv/h on the surface. Is there a reason to panic?
8. If the specific gamma constant of ^{137}Cs is 89.6 μSv/GBq-h, a compound unit at 1 m, calculate the dose at 40 cm from a 2.22 GBq source.
9. The specific gamma constant of ^{226}Ra is 222.8 μSv/GBq h at 1 m. What would the dose rate be at 50 cm from a 3.7 MBq source?
10. The gamma constant of ^{18}F is 154.7 μSv/GBq h at 1 m. What is the dose rate at 2 m from a 2-GBq source?

REFERENCES

Bevalacqua, J.J., *Basic Health Physics — Problems and Solutions*, Wiley–VCH, Weinheim, Germany, 1999.

Bouchet, L.G. et al., Considerations in the selection of radiopharmaceuticals for palliation of bone pain from metastatic osseous lesions, *J. Nucl. Med.*, 41, 682, 2000.

Chandra, R., *Nuclear Medicine Physics — The Basics*, 6th ed., Lippincott Williams & Wilkins, Philadelphia, 2004.

Chromic Phosphate P-32 Suspension, package insert, Mallinckrodt, Inc., St. Louis, 2000.

Dowd, S.B. and Tilson, E.R., *Practical Radiation Protection and Applied Radiobiology*, 2d ed., Saunders, Philadelphia, 1999.

Fiola, C., Monoclonal antibodies as anticancer agents, *U.S. Pharmacist*, 28, 1147, 2003.

Fluorodeoxyglucose F-18 Injection, package insert, Tampa PETNet Distribution Center, Tampa, 2005.

Goldsmith, S.J., Improving insight into radiobiology and radionuclide therapy, *J. Nucl. Med.*, 45, 1104, 2004.

Ibritumomab Tiuxetan, package insert, IDEC Pharmaceuticals Corporation, San Diego, 2002.

Iodine-131 Tositumomab, package insert, GlaxoSmithKline, Research Triangle Park, NC, 2005.

Koleskinov–Gautier, H. et al., Evaluation of toxicity and efficiency of ^{186}Re-hydroxy ethylidene diphosphonate in patients with painful bone metastases of prostatic and breast cancer, *J. Nucl. Med.*, 41, 1689, 2000.

Kowalsky, R.J. and Falen, S.W., *Radiopharmaceuticals in Nuclear Pharmacy and Nuclear Medicine*, 2d ed., American Pharmacists Association, Washington, DC, 2004.

Pandit–Taskar, N. et al., Radiopharmaceutical therapy for palliation of bone pain from osseous metastases, *J. Nucl. Med.*, 45, 1358, 2004.

Roberts, F.O. et al., Radiation dose to PET technologists and strategies to lower occupational dose, *J. Nucl. Med. Technol.*, 33, 44, 2005.

Saha, G.B., *Basics of PET Imaging*, Springer, New York, 2005.

Sandler, M.P. et al., Editors (Editors are Coleman, Patton, Wackers, and Gottschalk), *Diagnostic Nuclear Medicine*, Lippincott Williams & Wilkins, Philadelphia, 2003.

Sciuto, R. et al., Short and long-term effects of ^{186}Re-1-hydroxy ethylidene diphosphonate in the treatment of painful bone metatases, *J. Nucl. Med.*, 41, 647, 2000.

Shleien,B., Slaback, Jr., L.A., and Birky, B.K., Editors, *Handbook of Health Physics and Radiological Health*, 3d ed., Lippincott Williams & Wilkins, Philadelphia, 1998.

Silverstein, E.B. et al., SNM guidelines for palliative painful bone metastases, in *SNM Procedure Guidelines Manual*, Society of Nuclear Medicine, Reston, VA, 2003.

Silverstein, E.B., Radionuclides and radiopharmaceuticals for 2005, *J. Nucl. Med.*, 46, 13N, 2005.

Slater, R.J., *Radioisotopes in Biology*, 2d ed., Oxford University Press, Oxford, 2002.

Strontium-89 Chloride Injection, package insert, Medi-Physics, Inc., Arlington Heights, VA, 2000.

Thompson, M.A., Radiation safety precautions in the management of the hospitalized ^{131}I patient, *J. Nucl. Med.*, 29, 61, 2001.

Turner, J.E., Editor, *Atoms, Radiation, and Radiation Protection*, 2d ed., John Wiley & Sons, New York, 1995.

Wagner, H.N. et al., Administration guidelines for radioimmunotherapy of non-Hodgkins lymphoma with ^{90}Y-labeled anti-CD20 MoAb, *J. Nucl. Med.*, 43, 267, 2002.

Yttrium-90 Microspheres, package insert, Sirtex Medical, Inc., Lake Forest, IL, 2004.

Zimmerman, B.E. and Pipes, D.W., Experimental determination of dose calibrator settings and study associated volume dependence in V-vials for Rhenium-186 perrhenate solution sources, *J. Nucl Med.*, 28, 264, 2000.

7 Radiation Surveys and Waste Disposal

I. RATIONALE

The NM department is a very active place. Each day, as many as 500 mCi (18.5 GBq) of various radiopharmaceuticals are used in NM imaging procedures on some 50 patients. All those procedures must be done in a timely way while, at the same time, maintaining radiation safety. All staff members, physicians, technologists, and radiopharmacists must keep close attention to each step of every procedure to ensure the safety of the staff, patients, and visitors. First and foremost, they are their own safety officers because they must ensure their own safety in every task they perform, and second, they must ensure the safety of others.

Among the tasks that NMTs do everyday are (a) QA testing of imaging instrumentation, including PET/CT scanners, (b) QA testing of dose calibrators, (c) preparation of the needed RPs using kits, (d) QA of the imaging RPs, (e) assaying of multidosage vials with a dose calibrator, (f) dispensing of individual dosages for patients, (g) performing imaging procedures (data acquisition and processing), (h) printing of images and reports, and (i) submission of reports to physicians for interpretation. Upon completion of each task, all radioactive sources must be put away into shielded containers, cabinets, or refrigerators. And every disposable item that came into contact with radioactivity (vials, syringes, needles, swabs, paper tissues, gloves, etc.) must be disposed appropriately as radioactive waste.

To ascertain radiation safety, four goals must be accomplished: (a) on-time monitoring of all working areas of the NM department, (b) readiness of decontamination procedures should an accidental spill occur, (c) proper management of radioactive wastes, and (d) maintenance of records on all of the aforementioned. In this chapter, the basic procedures to accomplish those goals are described.

II. RADIATION SURVEYS

A. Preparation

The RSO or the designated person must (a) review the previous survey reports to identify previous problems, if any, (b) initiate a new survey report form, (c) identify sites of RP storage and use, (d) recognize sites of waste storage, (e) check shielded refrigerators, fume hoods, and glove boxes for proper operation, (f) identify the areas to be monitored and/or wipe-tested, (g) verify proper operation of survey instruments, including wipe counters, and (h) perform monitoring and wipe-testing as prescribed in the RSP.

B. Survey Practices

1. Proper selection of a survey instrument.
2. Proper calibration and operation of the selected instrument.
3. Correct use of instrument: shield cover for gamma, no cover for beta, thin window for weak beta radiation.
4. Where airborne radioactivity may be found, use of air monitors.
5. For tritium and carbon-14, wipe-testing, and liquid scintillation counting.
6. For low-level contamination or weak gamma rays, wipe-testing.
7. Routine wipe-testing of gamma cameras and other imaging instruments is recommended.

C. Selection of a Survey Instrument

To select a survey instrument, knowledge about the radionuclides involved and their emissions is essential. Knowing the level of activity used, the emission energies, and the tasks performed in each working area is imperative. Some examples follow:

1. In a compartment or area in which beta emitters are handled, a thin-window (1.4 mg/cm^2) GM survey meter would be needed.
2. Where millicurie amounts of pure-gamma emitters, such as ^{99m}Tc, are handled, a GM beta–gamma survey meter would suffice.
3. In a fume hood, where therapeutic dosages of ^{131}I are prepared, a GM beta–gamma survey meter should be chosen.
4. Similarly, in the imaging rooms, where ^{99m}Tc, ^{111}In, or ^{18}F are used, a GM beta–gamma survey meter would be quite appropriate.
5. In the radiopharmacy, where large quantities of radioactivity are handled daily, an ionization chamber should be chosen.
6. To check for the effectiveness of a decontamination procedure, a portable surface monitor would best do the job.
7. To measure the activity of wipes, a GM or a scintillation wipe counter should be used. Alternatively, a well-type gamma counter equipped with a single-channel or a multichannel analyzer could be used.

D. Proper Operation

1. Battery check: The instrument is turned on and set to “battery” at the lowest range setting. The meter should move to the battery range. If not, the batteries must be replaced. Some scintillation survey instruments require a “voltage” check before a survey can begin. Voltage can be adjusted to the proper range by turning a knob.

2. Performance check: Some instruments have a small ^{226}Ra or ^{137}Cs source to verify proper reading at a given distance. Follow the manufacturer's instructions.
3. Background check: Once the instrument is set for operation, a reading of background (bkg) must be taken in a "clean area" using the lowest scale. Usually bkg oscillates around 0.02 mR/h or 0.2 μSv/h.

E. Surveying of Working Areas

Routine department surveys are required and necessary to maintain safety (10CFR20.1501). They are mandated by the license, which specifies the frequency of surveys. All areas of the NM department are routinely surveyed. Special attention is given to the following:

1. The hot lab or radiopharmacy: Several monitorings per day are necessary because of the large amounts of radioactivity handled there. Some procedures done in the hot lab are preparation of RPs, QA of RPs, dispensing of imaging doses, elution of generators, assay of eluants, and QA of dose calibrators. Some patients may receive their RP dosages there.
2. Imaging rooms: Most patients receive their RP dosages in the imaging rooms just before the imaging procedure is to begin. Dosages may exceed 20 mCi (740 MBq) of ^{99m}Tc and 15 mCi (555 MBq) of ^{18}F.
3. Hospital rooms: Some patients are injected with the RP dosage in their hospital rooms, and later, they are brought to the NM department for the imaging procedure.
4. Nonimaging room: In this room, patients may receive 1 to10 μCi (37 to 370 kBq) of ^{131}I or 100 to 400 μCi (3.7 to 14.8 MBq) of ^{123}I for a thyroid uptake and/or imaging study.
5. The gamma counters room: This room is a low-level counting area. Because the detectors that measure patient samples are there, the area must be radioactively clean.

F. Methods

Routine surveys concern the following:

1. Survey meter monitoring: As scheduled, a portable GM beta–gamma survey meter is used to monitor all rooms, counters, tables, etc. See procedure below.
2. Wipe-test monitoring: Wipe-test monitoring is used to detect low levels and/or weak radiation contamination.
3. Leak-testing of sealed sources: Wipes or swabs are used to detect possible leakage of radioactivity from sealed sources. Testing is done at 6-month intervals; wipes must not contain more than 5 nCi (185 Bq) of removable radioactivity. See Chapter 5.

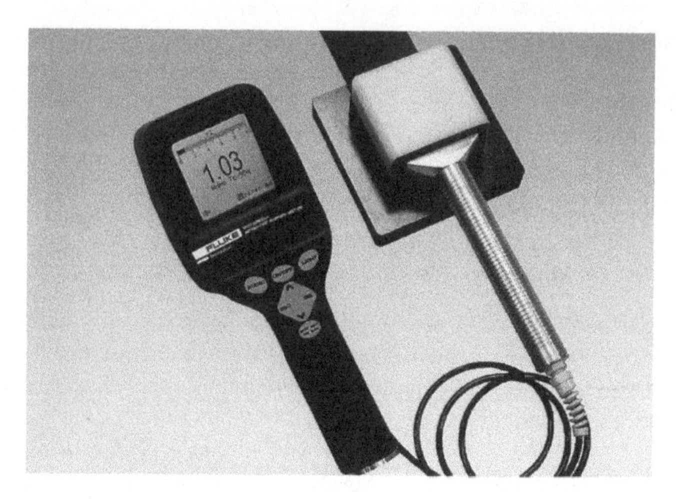

FIGURE 7.1 A high-efficiency scintillation survey meter. By changing detector probes, as shown, the instrument becomes a wipe-test measuring device for ^{99m}Tc surveys. (Courtesy of Fluke Biomedical, Cleveland, OH.)

III. SURVEY INSTRUMENTS

A. GM Survey Meters

These instruments are calibrated annually (10CFR20.1501). Calibration is done for all scales up to 1000 mR/h (10 mSv/h) by an authorized, licensed person. Calibration must be done for the low and high sides of each scale. A sticker on the side of the instrument must show any correction factors and the date of calibration. A certificate of calibration is placed on file. Records must be kept for three years (10CFR35.2061). Figure 7.1 shows a portable survey meter. By changing probes, the survey instrument becomes a wipe-testing device such as the one shown in the illustration.

B. Alarm Monitors

These instruments are bench-type GM counters placed in the hot lab or in some imaging rooms to monitor exposure rates continuously. An alarm sounds at a preset exposure rate, such as 15 or 20 mR/h (150 to 200 μSv/h). Figure 7.2 shows an alarm monitor specially designed for monitoring ^{133}Xe in the pulmonary ventilation room. This instrument is used to monitor air concentrations continuously. Results are expressed in DACs (derived air concentrations), or μCi/ml of air. When the DAC exceeds the set scale, the digital registers flash and an audible alarm is activated.

C. Ionization Chambers

As described in Chapter 4, these instruments can measure up to 50 R/h (500 mSv/h). For that reason, they are useful in hot labs and in commercial radiopharmacies.

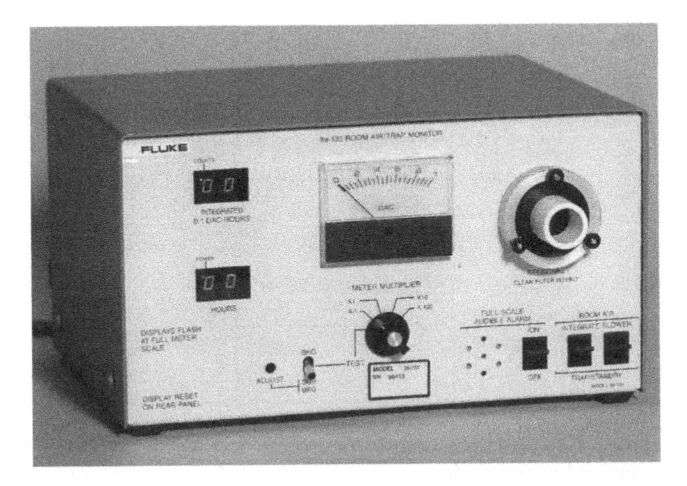

FIGURE 7.2 Alarm GM monitor specially designed for continuous air monitoring in the pulmonary ventilation room. (Courtesy of Fluke Biomedical, Cleveland, OH.)

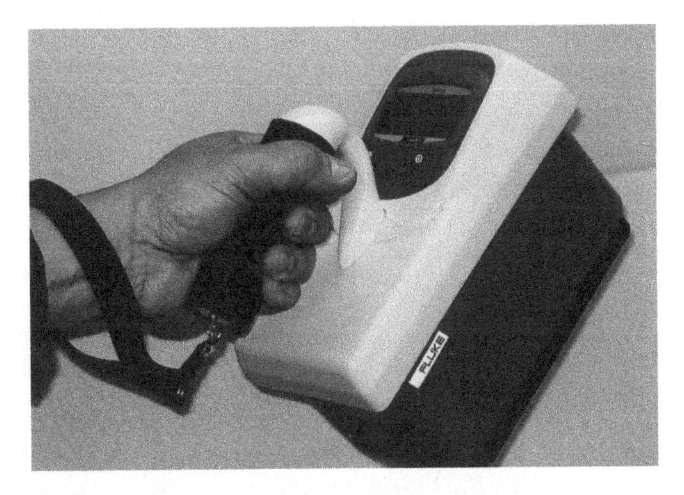

FIGURE 7.3 A state-of-the-art ionization chamber survey meter for monitoring of alpha, beta, gamma, and x-ray radiation. (Courtesy of Fluke Biomedical, Cleveland, OH.)

Figure 7.3 shows an ionization chamber survey meter for monitoring of alpha, beta, gamma, and x-ray radiations. The instrument has digital liquid crystal display (LCD), automatic zeroing, automatic scale ranging, and can be programmed for registers' flashing and for sounding an alarm.

D. Surface Monitors

These are specially designed instruments with a very thin window, designed to detect very low levels of contamination on floors, tables, counter tops, walls, etc. and to verify completion of decontamination.

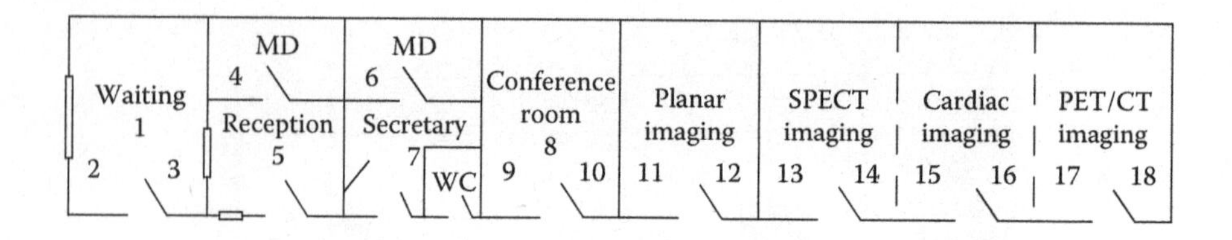

FIGURE 7.4 Map of an NM department showing symbolically 36 areas designated for routine monitoring and wipe-testing.

IV. MONITORING

A. Map of the Department

The RSO prepares a map of the department on which specific areas, instruments, benches, tables, etc., are designated by number for routine monitoring. Attached to the map is a chart where observed exposure rates are entered in addition to other pertinent information. Figure 7.4 is a sample of an NM department map.

B. Method

First, a background reading must be made in a "clean" area. The reading is entered on the chart. Table 7.1 is a sample of the chart. Second, all areas are monitored, and the readings are also entered on the chart. Any reading that exceeds the background plus three times its standard deviation is considered positive and must be monitored

TABLE 7.1
Radiation Survey Record

Date ________	Instrument ________	Bkg. Range ________	
Areas	1. ______ mR/h	13. ______ mR/h	25. ______ mR/h
	2. ______	14. ______	26. ______
	3. ______	15. ______	27. ______
	....	....	....
	12. ______	24. ______	36. ______

Comments:

Signature: ____________________________

again and wipe-tested. Another practical approach is that any reading that is twice the mean background is positive and must be wipe-tested.

C. Hot-Lab Housekeeping

In addition to continuous alarm monitoring and frequent surveying, covering all work areas with absorbent paper with impermeable backing is absolutely essential. The paper is replaced frequently.

D. Wipe-Test Monitoring

1. This method of monitoring is an efficient way of detecting any low-level or low-energy radioactivities, in the nonimaging room, in the gamma counters room, and in the imaging rooms.
2. Commércially available or homemade disks of absorbent paper are numbered according to the areas to be monitored routinely (Figure 7.4). Wearing gloves, the assigned person wipes each area with the corresponding disk. Wiping is done in a circular motion of about 11.3 cm (4.4 inches) in diameter for an area of 100 cm^2 or 20 cm (8 in.) in diameter for an area of about 300 cm^2.
3. Wipes are placed in test tubes and measured for radioactivity in a well-type scintillation gamma counter or in a wipe-test counter. If using a gamma counter, countings are done setting windows for the main peaks of the gamma spectrum of ^{99m}Tc, ^{111}In, ^{133}Xe, ^{67}Ga, ^{131}I, ^{125}I, or ^{18}F, as the case may be. Figure 7.1 shows a high-efficiency scintillation detector for ^{99m}Tc wipes.
4. Net count rates can be converted into DPMs (disintegrations per minute) using a suitable standard. Any wipe containing more than 6,600 DPM/300 cm^2 or 2,200 DPM/100 cm^2 is considered positive. This values correspond respectively to 3 nCi and 1 nCi of removable radioactivity.
5. Table 7.2 is an example of a report form used to record wipe-test results.

TABLE 7.2
Wipe-Test Survey Record

Date ________ Instrument ________ Bkg. ________ c/min

Areas	1. ______ c/min	13. ______ c/min	25. ______ c/min
	2. ______	14. ______	26. ______
	3. ______	15. ______	27. ______
	....	....	....
	12. ______	24. ______	36. ______

Comments:

Signature: ____________________

V. ACCIDENTAL CONTAMINATION

A. Radioactive Spills

Radioactive spills can occur in a very busy NM department. For example,

1. Radioactive solutions can spill in transit, inside containers, during preparation, during QA testing, while loading syringes, or while injecting patients. Keen concentration by the staff is essential at all times to prevent accidental spills and accidental needle stings. Follow hospital policy regarding needle stings.
2. Radioactive gases, such as ^{133}Xe, can be released accidentally during the administration of a dosage to a patient. Working in the fume hood, using dedicated dispensing systems, and rehearsing the procedure before administration, etc., can prevent accidental releases of the radioactive gas.
3. Radioactive sealed sources can be misplaced, can be stolen, or may leak. Doing inventories and leak-tests as scheduled can prevent losses and unnecessary exposures.

B. Decontamination

1. Minor Spills

Minor spills represent the release of several microcuries (over 100 kBq) of radioactivity. They could occur in the nonimaging procedures room, in the gamma counters room, or in the imaging rooms. The person involved (a) warns other workers, (b) wearing gloves, proceeds to decontaminate the area immediately, (c) informs the RSO, and (d) has the RSO prepare an incident report for the files.

2. Major Spills

Major spills involve the release of several millicuries (over 100 MBq) of radioactivity. They could occur in the hot lab, the imaging rooms, or the radionuclide therapy room. The person involved warns other radiation workers, closes the area to traffic, and summons the RSO who immediately assesses the situation and gives directions for decontamination. Figure 7.5 shows a sample of a kit used in the process of decontamination. The items shown are assembled on an emergency cart ready to go to the site of a major spill. A guide follows:

a. An assessment of the quality and quantity of radioactivity spilled is made. The area covered by the spill is recognized by monitoring. If any worker is injured, medical assistance is requested immediately.
b. The RSO brings the emergency cart and places appropriate radiation warning signs, such as "CAUTION — RADIOACTIVE CONTAMINATION." Using a portable survey meter, exposure rates are determined.
c. If any worker is contaminated, removal of contaminated clothes and showering may be necessary. Contaminated clothes, shoes, etc. are placed

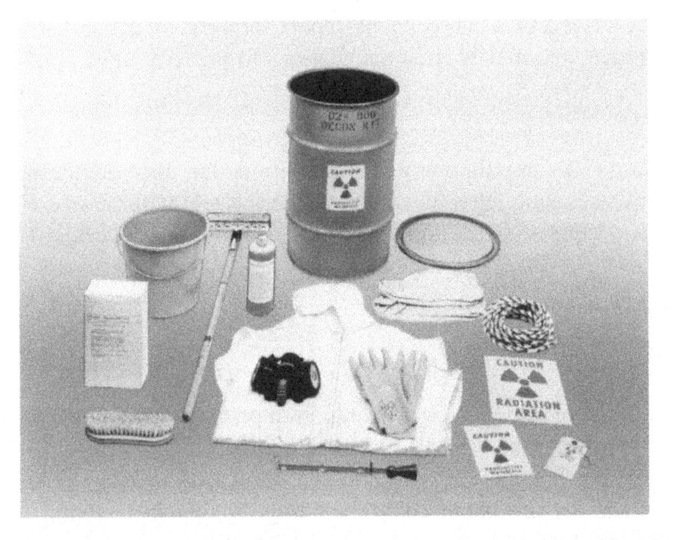

FIGURE 7.5 Decontamination kit. Warning signs, rope to restrict traffic, cleaning tools and solutions, mask, gloves, shoe covers, and other items are shown. (Courtesy of Fluke Biomedical, Cleveland, OH.)

in a plastic bag for decay in storage. Flushing the eyes with water may be necessary. After showering, monitoring is done to confirm complete decontamination.

d. In case of fire, an attempt to put out the fire must be done immediately while someone calls for the fire emergency units.

3. Procedure

a. Wearing protective clothing, a disposable laboratory coat, gloves, and shoe covers, the worker proceeds to pick up most of the spilled solution with absorbent paper towels held with 18-in. forceps.
b. The pickup procedure is the "spiral-in technique:" the contaminated area is wiped with paper towels starting at the periphery and in a circular motion toward the center of the area. The wet towels are placed in double plastic bags.
c. Any broken glass is carefully picked up and placed in hard plastic or metal containers.
d. Cleaning solutions are then used to decontaminate the area. Repeated cleaning may be needed. Refer to Schleien's Handbook, pages 11–92.
e. Monitoring of the area with a surface monitor will confirm complete decontamination: less than 2 mR/h (0.2 μSv/h).
f. Plastic bags containing radioactivity are placed in a large metal drum lined with a heavy-duty plastic bag. The cylinder is labeled and sent to decay in storage. Records are entered in the waste disposal logbook. All disposable gloves, shoe covers, etc., are disposed as contaminated.

g. The RSO prepares an incident report, reports to the radiation safety committee, and makes recommendations to prevent future spills.

C. Release of ^{133}Xe

Licensees using ^{133}Xe in pulmonary ventilation imaging must demonstrate by measurement or by calculation that they do not exceed the DAC limit of 1×10^{-4} μCi/ml of air (3.7×10^{-3} kBq/ml) in the pulmonary ventilation room. An example calculation follows.

Sample Problem

Assume that

a. An average of 100 pulmonary ventilation procedures are done per month.
b. In each procedure, 370 MBq are used/patient.
c. The air flow in the room is 400 ft^3/min, equivalent to 1.132×10^7 ml/min.
d. That there are just about 10,000 working minutes in 1 month.
e. In the worst possible scenario, 10% of the ^{133}Xe gas is released.

It follows that

$$^{133}\text{Xe used: } 370 \text{ MBq/patient} \times 100 \text{ pts/month} = 3.7 \times 10^4 \text{ MBq/month}$$
$$^{133}\text{Xe released: } 10\% \text{ of } 3.7 \times 10^4 \text{ MBq/month} = 3.7 \times 10^3 \text{ MBq/month}$$
$$= 3.7 \times 10^{-1} \text{ MBq/min}$$
$$= 370 \text{ kBq/min}$$

Dividing 370 kBq/min by 1.132 ml/min = 3.27×10^{-3} kBq/ml of air, which is less than the DAC limit for ^{133}Xe. See also Table 3.2.

VI. RADIOACTIVE WASTES

The NM department in hospitals and clinics does not produce significant amounts of radioactive waste. Essentially, all the waste is converted into nonradioactive waste by decay in storage (DIS). However, the industries that supply hospitals with radionuclide generators and other radiopharmaceuticals do produce significant amounts of radioactive waste. Thus, directly or indirectly, the problem of radioactive wastes concerns all in the practice of NM.

A. Classes of Radioactive Wastes

1. *High-level wastes* (HLW): These are the remnants in the processing and reprocessing of nuclear reactor fuels. Those fuels are used in the nuclear power industry.
2. *Spent reactor fuel* (SRF): These are fuel assembly units in storage at reactor facilities awaiting disposal.
3. *Transuranic wastes* (TRU): Wastes produced during the production of plutonium-239 in the nuclear weapons industry.

4. *Low-level wastes* (LLW): Waste produced by all radioisotope production, purification, and applications, including biomedical research at governmental installations and universities, production of radiopharmaceuticals by private industry, and NM practice at hospitals and clinics.

B. Nuclear Medicine Wastes

NM wastes fall in the category of LLWs. Most of the radioactive materials used in hospitals and clinics are short-lived, with half-lives under 120 d. As authorized by 10CFR35.92, they can be allowed to decay in storage (DIS) and then be disposed as nonradioactive wastes. Agencies concerned with the packaging and shipment of radioactive wastes are the NRC, the DOT, and the FAA (federal aviation agency). See other agencies in the following text.

1. Solid Wastes

Solid wastes consist of used hypodermic syringes, needles, alcohol wipes, cotton balls, disposable gloves, used absorbent paper, used RP vials, paper towels, used gauze pads, paper tissues, empty plastic containers of various kinds, etc. Those items that contain, or came in contact with, patients' body fluids are classified as biohazards and, therefore, may require sterilization before disposal. Refer to hospital policy.

2. Liquid Wastes

Leftover samples of blood, serum, plasma, urine, etc. in test tubes and other containers are biohazards and may require sterilization by physical or chemical means before incineration. Recommended hospital epidemiology procedures should be followed. Other liquid wastes are leftover radioactive solutions such as generator eluants and other RP remnants in glass vials.

3. Radioactive Gases

Although the radiopharmaceutical industry formulates radioiodine solutions to minimize volatilization, minute quantities of ^{125}I, ^{123}I, and ^{131}I could be released into the air. For that reason, all radioiodine work should be done in a properly functioning fume hood or glove box equipped with sodium hydroxide traps or other means of reducing airborne radioactivity. During pulmonary ventilation imaging, the accidental release of ^{133}Xe or ^{99m}Tc-DTPA aerosol is possible. The use of closed dispensing systems can prevent accidental releases. For ^{133}Xe, the gas used can be trapped in charcoal canisters within a shielded box.

C. Radiotoxicity

Radiotoxicity is the disruption of life functions due to the radiation energy deposition in cells and tissues. According to their radiotoxicity, most NM radionuclides fall into three groups:

1. High toxicity: ^{90}Sr, ^{125}I, and ^{131}I.
2. Moderate toxicity: ^{14}C, ^{18}F, ^{33}P, ^{57}Co, ^{58}Co, ^{89}Sr, ^{90}Y, ^{99}Mo, ^{123}I, ^{153}Sm, ^{186}Re, ^{188}Re, and ^{201}Tl.
3. Low toxicity: ^{15}O, ^{99m}Tc, ^{129}I, and ^{133}Xe.

VII. DISPOSAL OF RADIOACTIVE WASTES

A. Disposal of Solid Wastes

The radiopharmacist or the person assigned to the hot lab plays a key role in the housekeeping of the laboratory, the management of wastes, and the maintenance of ALARA.

1. Management of Wastes (10CFR20.2001)

Radioactive wastes with half-lives under 120 d are allowed to decay in storage (DIS) before disposal as nonradioactive (10CFR35.92). The management of wastes involves (a) segregation of wastes into classes by type and half-life, (b) temporary storage in shielded cabinets in the hot lab, and (c) their submission to DIS. Verification of complete decay is done ten half-lives later followed by disposal as nonradioactive waste. Finally, the maintenance of accurate records on all of the above tasks is required. Records are to be maintained for a minimum of three years.

2. Segregation by Half-Life

a. Hours: ^{99m}Tc, ^{123}I, ^{18}F, ^{188}Re, ^{11}C, ^{13}N, ^{15}O, ^{68}Ga, and ^{82}Rb.
b. Days: ^{133}Xe, ^{201}Tl, ^{67}Ga, ^{99}Mo, ^{111}In, ^{186}Re, ^{153}Sm, and ^{90}Y.
c. Weeks: ^{131}I, ^{51}Cr, ^{125}I, ^{32}P, ^{59}Fe, ^{57}Co, ^{89}Sr, ^{177}Lu, and ^{90}Sr.

3. Biohazards

Any item that came in contact with a patient's body fluids may have to be sterilized before incineration. Follow hospital policy.

4. Radiopharmaceutical Remnants

Vials containing small amounts of RP remnants are classified by half-life, placed in plastic bags, labeled, and stored temporarily in shielded cabinets in the hot lab. Later in the day, they are transferred to storage drums in the DIS room.

5. Nuclide Generators

By the end of the week, ^{99m}Tc generators still contain 50 or more mCi of ^{99}Mo. They can be allowed to DIS or, by agreement, returned to the supplier in their original containers. If radioactive, follow U.S. DOT shipping regulations. Other RP lead containers may follow the same steps as generators or may be disposed as scrap metal. Follow hospital policy.

TABLE 7.3
Effluent Concentration Limits

Radionuclide	Air (μCi/ml)	Water (μCi/ml)	Sewer (μCi/ml)
^{131}I	2×10^{-10}	1×10^{-6}	1×10^{-5}
^{125}I	3×10^{-10}	2×10^{-6}	2×10^{-5}
^{133}Xe	5×10^{-7}	—	—
^{99m}Tc	3×10^{-7}	1×10^{-3}	1×10^{-2}
^{18}F	1×10^{-7}	7×10^{-4}	7×10^{-3}

6. Labeling

All containers with radioactive waste must be labeled with their contents, date, initials, and warning signs (10CFR35.69). Warning signs must also be placed on the door of the DIS room. Accessibility to the DIS room is allowed to authorized persons only.

7. Records

Every time wastes are sent to the DIS room, the radionuclides, their amounts, the dates, etc., are also entered in the "Radioactive Wastes" logbook kept in the hot lab ready for inspection. Records must be kept for three years.

B. Liquid Wastes Disposal

Regulations allow the disposal of small amounts of liquid radioactivity through the "hot sink" in the hot lab (10CFR35.2003). This hot waste must be soluble or readily dispersible in water. These releases affect the general public. The monthly average concentration cannot exceed the effluent concentration limits shown in Table 7.3. The total yearly release cannot exceed 1 Ci (37 GBq). Accurate records must be kept as indicated for DIS. Because most of the liquid waste can be converted into solid waste by adding absorbent paper or other absorbent material, and then be allowed to DIS, there is no real reason for disposal through the hot sink. RP remnants in vials with rubber closures are placed in plastic bags and sent to DIS. Patients' excreta are exempted from these regulations.

C. Gases, Aerosols, and Volatile Radioiodine

Multiple dose vials of ^{133}Xe are stored in their original containers. After drawing the first dose, they must be stored in the fume hood. During pulmonary ventilation studies, the room must have a ventilation system that allows negative pressure with regard to the immediate halls or rooms. The room door must be closed, and the gas/aerosol must be dispensed using an airtight closed system. Under these conditions, by calculation, it can be demonstrated that accidental releases of ^{133}Xe gas are inconsequential. Reminder: the biological half-life of ^{133}Xe in normal individuals is approximately 20 seconds. See also the section titled "Release of ^{133}Xe" earlier in this chapter. Table 7.3 shows the NRC concentration limits for releases into the air.

There is a potential for volatilization of ^{131}I and ^{125}I from their solutions. For that reason, they must be handled in a properly operating fume hood and behind shielding. They can be absorbed through the skin. For that reason, wearing gloves is imperative. The use of syringe shields is strongly recommended.

D. Transportation of Wastes

Agencies concerned with the transportation of radioactive wastes are the NRC, the DOE, the DOT, the U.S. Postal Service, the U.S. Coast Guard, the Federal Aviation Agency, and the state government agencies.

VIII. OCCUPATIONAL EXPOSURES

A. Occupational Exposure to ^{131}I

The licensee must demonstrate by either measurement or calculation that the staff is not exposed to ^{131}I in the drinkable water or air in the NM department in quantities exceeding the annual limits on intake (ALIs), which for ^{131}I are

90 μCi in drinkable water
50 μCi in the thyroid gland from air
200 μCi in the whole body from air

The derived air concentration (DAC) that, in the average worker, would result in the ALIs shown above is 2×10^{-8} μCi/ml of air. See Table 3.2.

B. Occupational Exposure to ^{133}Xe

Xenon-133 is obtained in gaseous form contained in sealed vials. It is never found in drinkable water. The biological half-life is about 20 seconds. No ALIs have been listed. However, the DAC has been set at 1×10^{-4} μCi/mL of air. Licensees must demonstrate that such DAC is never reached in the NM department. See the calculation earlier in this chapter.

IX. THE ENVIRONMENTAL PROTECTION AGENCY (EPA)

The EPA regulation 40CFR61.I sets limits for radionuclide emissions into the air, which apply to commercial radiopharmacies as well as NM departments of hospitals and clinics. The EPA limits radionuclide emissions to amounts that would not result in more than 10 mrem/y (100 μSv/y) of equivalent dose to any member of the public. Of those 10 mrem, no more than 3 mrem (30 μSv) can be due to radioiodine.

1. These limits are more restrictive than those of the NRC, which sets the yearly individual dose to the public at 100 mrem/y (1 mSv/y) from all sources.

2. The basis for the EPA limits is the risk of cancer, which for 10 mrem (100 μSv) represents one excess cancer per 10,000 persons/y of the general public.
3. Specific EPA concentration limits for releases into the air are

$$^{131}\text{I}: 2.1 \times 10^{-13}\ \mu\text{Ci/ml}\ (7.77 \times 10^{-12}\ \text{kBq/ml})$$

$$^{133}\text{Xe}: 6.2 \times 10^{-8}\ \mu\text{Ci/ml}\ (2.29 \times 10^{-6}\ \text{kBq/ml})$$

4. Medical institutions must, by calculation or measurement, demonstrate compliance with EPA regulations and file a yearly report.
5. Most NM departments do not use radioiodine or ^{133}Xe in quantities that require reporting to the EPA. The use of fume hoods, radioiodine traps, and airtight ^{133}Xe dispensing systems facilitates compliance. Continuous monitoring of nonrestricted areas in the NM department with thermoluminescent dosimeters (TLD) can demonstrate compliance.

PROBLEMS

Problems in this chapter concern occupational and nonoccupational dose limits.

1. What are the annual occupational dose limits for the lenses of the eyes?
2. What are the annual occupational dose limits for the whole-body skin?
3. At what depth of the body is the shallow equivalent dose defined?
4. What is the dose limit to the human fetus during gestation?
5. According to the NCRP, is 10 mrem (100 μSv) a negligible dose?
6. What is the annual dose limit for the hands of a radiation worker?
7. What is the annual dose limit to the whole body of a technologist?
8. What are the specific gamma constants for ^{99}Mo and ^{99m}Tc?
9. What is the annual EPA dose limit for individuals of the general public from radioactivity releases into the air?
10. What is the risk of cancer that corresponds to the EPA dose limit of Problem 9?

REFERENCES

Bevalacqua, J.J., *Basic Health Physics — Problems and Solutions*, Wiley–VCH, Weinheim, Germany, 1999.

Code of Federal Regulations, Title 10, National Archives and Records Administration, Washington, DC, 2005.

Chandra, R., *Nuclear Medicine Physics — The Basics*, 6th ed., Lippincott Williams & Wilkins, Philadelphia, 2004.

Dowd, S.B. and Tilson, E.R., *Practical Radiation Protection and Applied Radiobiology*, 2d ed., Saunders, Philadelphia, 1999.

Early, P.J., *Review of Rules and Regulations Governing the Practice of Nuclear Medicine*, 41st Annual Meeting of the Society of Nuclear Medicine, Orlando, 1994.

Fluke Biomedical, Radiation Management Services Product Catalog, Cleveland, 2005.

Gallo Foss, A.M., *Review Questions for Nuclear Medicine — The Technology Registry Examination*, The Parthenon Publishing Group, New York, 1997.

Guillet, B. et al., Technologist radiation exposure in routine clinical practice with ^{18}FDG PET, *J. Nucl. Med. Technol.*, 33, 175, 2005.

Kane, D.F., The clean air act and nuclear medicine, *J. Nucl. Med. Technol.*, 24 (1), 1996.

Kasner, D.L. and Spieth, M.E., The day of contamination, *J. Nucl. Med. Technol.*, 31, 21, 2003.

Lundberg, T.M. et al., Measuring and minimizing radiation dose to nuclear medicine technologists, *J. Nucl. Med. Technol.*, 30, 25, 2002.

Mason, J.S., Elliot K.M., and Mitro, A.C., *The Nuclear Medicine Handbook for Achieving Compliance with NRC Regulations*, Society of Nuclear Medicine, Reston, VA, 1997.

Noz, M.E. and Maguire, G.Q., *Radiation Protection in the Radiologic and Health Sciences*, 3d ed., Lea & Febiger, Philadelphia, 1995.

Nuclear Energy Low-Level Radioactive Wastes, American Nuclear Society, La Grange Park, IL, 1993.

Performance and Responsibility Guidelines for Nuclear Medicine Technologists, Society of Nuclear Medicine, Technology Section, Reston, VA, 2003.

Roberts, F.O. et al., Radiation dose to PET technologists and strategies to lower occupational dose, *J. Nucl. Med. Technol.*, 33, 44, 2005.

Saha, G.B., *Physics and Radiobiology of Nuclear Medicine*, Springer–Verlag, New York, 1993.

Saha, G.B., *Basics of PET Imaging*, Springer, New York, 2005.

Sandler, M.P. et al., Editors (Coleman, Patton, Wackers, and Gottschalk), *Diagnostic Nuclear Medicine*, Lippincott Williams & Wilkins, Philadelphia, 2003.

Schelbert, H.R. et al., *SNM Procedure Guideline for Tumor Imaging Using F-18 FDG*, Society of Nuclear Medicine, Reston, VA, 1999.

Shleien, B., Slaback, Jr., L.A., and Birky, B.K., *Handbook of Health Physics and Radiological Health*, 3d ed., Lippincott Williams & Wilkins, Philadelphia, 1998.

Steves, A.M., *Review of Nuclear Medicine Technology*, 2d ed., Society of Nuclear Medicine, Reston, VA, 1996.

Tsopelas, C. et al., A simple and effective technique to reduce staff exposure during preparation of radiopharmaceuticals, *J. Nucl. Med. Technol.* 31, 37, 2003.

8 Monitoring of Personnel Exposures

I. RATIONALE

In the NM department, most personnel exposures are external. Internal exposures can be easily prevented by applying basic rules of safety. External exposures occur during (a) elution of nuclide generators, (b) assay of eluants, (c) preparation of radiopharmaceuticals (RPs), (d) dispensing of patients' dosages, (e) injection of RPs, (f) performance of imaging procedures, and (g) handling of radioactive wastes.

Most of the external doses received are due to gamma radiation. Secondarily, x-rays may represent some significant exposure for workers who use ^{201}Tl and ^{125}I. Beta radiation exposure is a real risk to persons working on radionuclide therapy. Beta radiation is also incidental to ^{133}Xe and ^{131}I. Conversion electrons are present in ^{99m}Tc and ^{125}I, and ^{201}Tl and ^{117m}Sn emissions. And, let us not forget that PET imaging agents are beta emitters. To reduce external exposures, radiation workers must practice radiation safety, i.e., the effective use of distance, shielding, and time. They must also minimize exposures by practicing ALARA.

The use of protective equipment plays an important role in this regard: long-sleeved laboratory coats, lead–glass goggles, disposable gloves, lead–glass windows on vial shields and lead syringe shields, lead storage containers, tungsten syringe shields, lead–glass barriers, lead–brick enclosures, forceps, tongs, and timers are essential to the safe handling of radiopharmaceuticals. Some of those protective devices are specially designed for PET procedures, and others are specially designed for radionuclide therapy.

Practicing radiation safety is not sufficient. The actual exposure of each individual radiation worker must be measured and documented using a certified monitoring procedure. Thus, radiopharmacists, nuclear medicine technologists (NMTs), and nuclear MDs must be continuously monitored for whole-body exposure. Individuals who elute generators, prepare, dispense, or inject radiopharmaceuticals must wear a hand dosimeter to measure and record the extremity dose. Fetal-dose monitoring is also required for declared pregnancies. In this chapter, the requirements, methods, reporting, and maintenance of records of personnel exposures are presented and discussed.

II. MONITORING OF OCCUPATIONAL EXPOSURES

A. Dose Limits

Part 20, Title 10 of the U.S. Code of Federal Regulations (10CFR20) sets dose limits for workers who use by-product materials only. Most states, by agreement, have accepted application of the limits to all radioactivities used, including accelerator-produced radionuclides such as ^{201}Tl, ^{67}Ga, ^{123}I, ^{111}In, ^{18}F, ^{11}C, ^{13}N, and ^{15}O, among others.

B. Requirements

1. Whole-body exposure monitoring is required for any worker who is likely to receive 10% of the occupational dose limit.
2. The same is required for any visitor entering a high-radiation area: more than 100 mrem/h (1 mSv/h), not likely in an NM department.
3. The licensee is also required to assess the committed effective dose E(τ) for any worker who is likely to receive 10% of the annual limit on intake (ALI).
4. Also required is the monitoring of doses received by minors visiting the department.
5. Embryo or fetal monitoring of any declared pregnancy among the staff is required.

Staff members in the NM department who must be monitored for whole-body exposure are NMTs, radiopharmacists, nuclear MDs, medical physicists, and some ancillary personnel such as patient transporters and nurses caring for radionuclide therapy patients.

III. REMINDER OF DOSE LIMITS

A. Occupational Dose Limits (10CFR20.1201)

Effective equivalent dose, whole-body	5 rem/y	(50 mSv/y)
Cumulative whole-body dose	1 rem × age	(10 mSv × age)
Lens equivalent dose	15 rem/y	(150 mSv/y)
Skin, hands, and feet	50 rem/y	(500 mSv/y)
Declared pregnancy	50 mrem/month	(500 μSv/month)

B. Nonoccupational Dose Limits (10CFR20.1301)

Whole-body, continuous exposure	100 mrem/y	(1 mSv/y)
Whole-body, infrequent exposure	500 mrem/y	(5 mSv/y)
Lens equivalent dose	1.5 rem/y	(15 mSv/y)
Skin, hands, and feet	5 rem/y	(50 mSv/y)
Minors in training (under 18 y)	10% of occupational dose	

The licensee must demonstrate that non-restricted areas, which are accessible to the general public, comply with nonoccupational dose limits. Those areas are the waiting room, the reception office, and the clerical offices. Film badge or thermoluminescence dosimetry (TLD) dosimeters, placed in some locations in those areas for continuous monitoring, can demonstrate compliance "by measurement." Dosimeters are sent to the service provider for reading and documenting. Dosimeters are changed monthly.

Dose limits in nonrestricted areas are 2 mrem/h (0.02 mSv/h) and 100 mrem/y (1 mSv/y).

IV. MONITORING METHODS

A. Acceptable Methods

1. Regulations require that the monitoring method used be accredited by the National Voluntary Laboratory Accreditation Program (NVLAP) of the National Institute of Standards and Technology (10CFR20.1501). At present, several commercial agencies provide this service to hospitals and clinics under contract.
2. Whole-body-monitoring methods are
   a. *Film badge method*: Uses x-ray film inside a special case
   b. *TLD badges*: Uses thermoluminescence dosimeters
   c. *Pocket dosimeters*: Pen-size ionization chamber detectors
   d. *Personal alarm monitors*: Require a reliable recording method
   e. *OSL*: Optically stimulated luminescence
3. Hand-dose-monitoring methods are
   a. *TLD ring dosimeters*: Worn on the preferred hand
   b. *Film badges*: Placed on the wrist of the preferred hand
   c. *Pocket dosimeters*: Placed on the wrists of both hands

B. Film Badge Dosimetry

1. The Service

Hospitals and clinics contract the service from a commercial agency. The badge cases are provided for all users initially. Thereafter, films are changed monthly. Personnel-exposure records are sent to the customer by the service provider monthly. With each monthly batch of films, the provider sends a "control" film to be kept in an unexposed place at the customer's facility. Control films are returned with the rest of the films for processing. Badges are to be worn on the laboratory coat at the level (collar, chest, or waist) closest to the sources handled.

2. The Badge Case

This is a device made of plastic material to hold the x-ray film in its sealed, impermeable envelope. The case has an open window, three different thicknesses of plastic, and two metal filters of aluminum and lead. These serve as attenuators

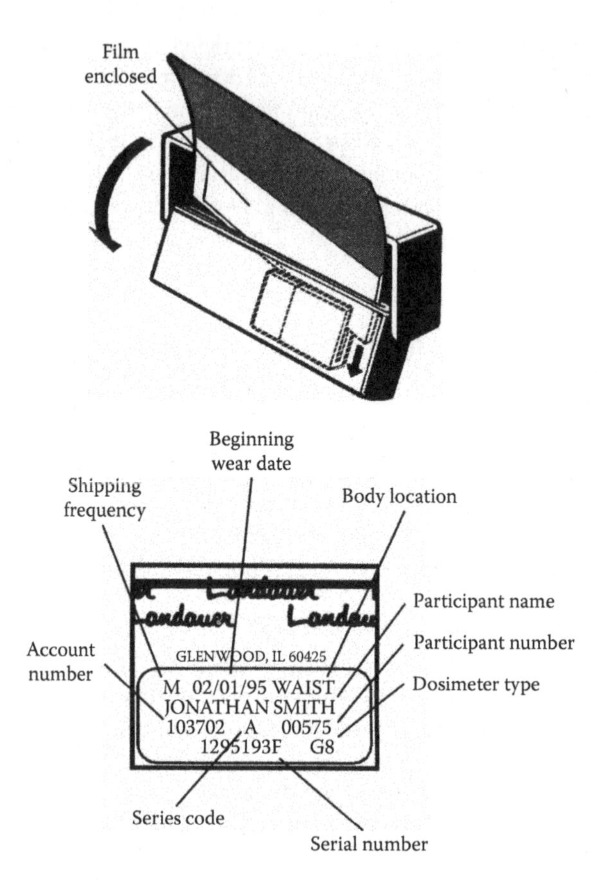

FIGURE 8.1 Film and film badge showing the metallic filters inside (top). Film envelope showing the method of identification (bottom). (Courtesy of Landauer, Inc., Glenwood, IL.)

to distinguish weak beta rays, strong beta rays, low-energy photons, and high-energy photons. A total of six areas on the film are read, and calculations are made to arrive at the wearer's doses. Figure 8.1 shows a film badge case and the method of film identification.

3. The Film

The film used is x-ray sensitive, dental-type, made of cellulose acetate coated on both sides with photographic emulsion 12 μm thick. The two sides have emulsions of different sensitivities. The total thickness is 0.2 mm. The film itself is coded for identification. The film is placed in a sealed envelope on which data relevant to identification and date are printed.

4. The Emulsion

The photographic emulsion is made of a gelatin base containing silver bromide (AgBr) crystals 0.2 to 2 μm in size.

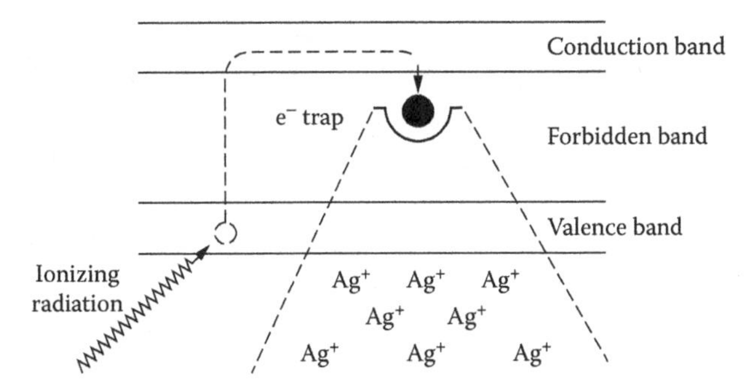

FIGURE 8.2 Diagram of a silver bromide crystal in the photographic emulsion. Electrons trapped in the forbidden band act as condensation centers for silver ions. Ion clusters make up the grains in the latent image.

5. The Theory

Gamma-ray or x-ray photons interact by photoelectric effect with electrons of the valence band on the AgBr crystals (Figure 8.2). In the process, the electrons are raised to the conduction band, where they roam free. Soon, they fall into crystal imperfections called *electron traps*. In that position, they act as "condensation centers" for silver ions. Clusters of silver ions make up the "grains" of the latent image.

6. Film Processing

Briefly, during development of the film, at 68°F (20°C), and under a safe light, the latent image is revealed. Rinsing and fixing of the "image" follows. This step removes the unused AgBr from the film. The concentration of grains is directly proportional to the radiation dose received. An infinite number of shades of gray is possible. The degree of grayness is known as *density*.

7. Density

The density of the film is directly related to the radiation exposure received during the month the badge was worn by the user. The filters in the badge case allow recognition of the types of radiations and measurement of the quantities of radiations that exposed the film during the month. The density is measured with a "densitometer." Briefly, a collimated beam of light of a given intensity (I_0) is shone through the film. On the opposite side, a light diode converts the transmitted light intensity (I_t) to an electrical current proportional to its density. Figure 8.3 shows a diagram of a densitometer. Basic concepts of film dosimetry are

a. Transmittance (T) = I_t/I_0
b. Opacity = I_0/I_t
c. Density (D) = log of opacity

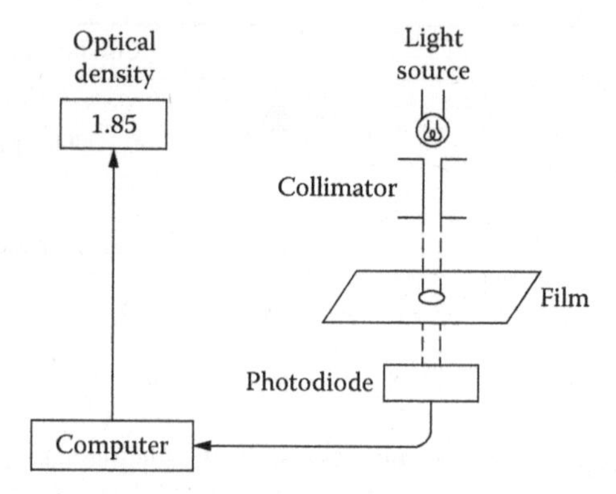

FIGURE 8.3 Diagram of a densitometer. A collimated beam of light passes through the film. The transmitted light is converted into an electrical signal by a photodiode. A microchip calculates the display densities.

8. Calibration Curve

To convert density into radiation dose, a calibration curve must be prepared with each batch of films. The curve is also known as the *H & D curve* for Hutter and Driffield, the scientists who first described it. The densitometer is set at zero with the control film and a separate set of films, exposed to accurate doses from an NBS-certified radiation source, are also read. A computer plots the densities as a function of dose. Using the data of the curve, the computer also calculates and prints doses for each user in the batch. Figure 8.4 shows a sample of an H & D curve. Characteristics of the curve shown are the following:

a. Shape of an italic "S."
b. Wide range of doses.
c. Insensitive below 10 mrem (100 μSv).
d. Insensitive above 100 rem (1 Sv).

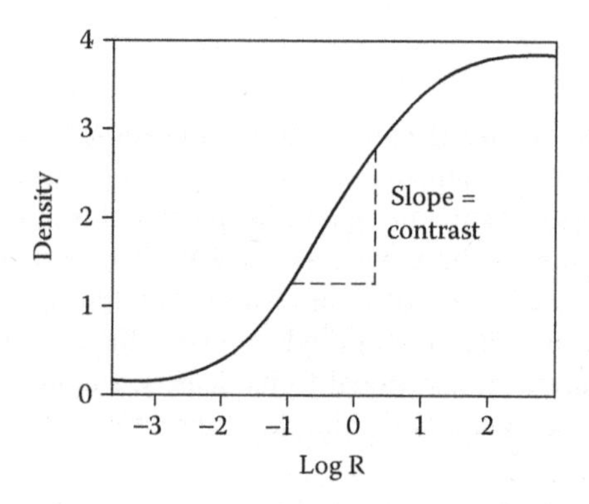

FIGURE 8.4 The H & D curve of an x-ray film. A linear graph of densities vs. the known radiation doses from a certified source.

e. The central portion of the curve is the *useful range.*
f. The slope of the curve is known as *contrast.*
g. For each batch of films, an H & D curve must be prepared.

9. Advantages

Film badge services are inexpensive and provide a permanent record. Films can be reread if necessary. The method is qualitative and quantitative. The method is reproducible, and the NRC and other licensing agencies recognize it and accept it.

10. Disadvantages

Films are affected by high temperatures (fogging). The quality assurance testing of the procedure must be very strict to maintain high standards of performance. A calibration curve must be prepared for each batch. Turnover time is about 4 to 6 weeks.

C. Thermoluminescence Dosimetry (TLD)

1. The Principle

The word *thermoluminescence* means emission of light upon heating, which is a property of certain substances such as lithium fluoride (LiF) or calcium fluoride (CaF_2). When their crystals are exposed to gamma or x-rays and then heated, they emit flashes of light. The intensity of the light emitted is proportional to the absorbed radiation dose.

2. The Theory

Figure 8.5 shows a diagram of an LiF crystal. The X- or gamma rays interact by photoelectric effect with electrons in the valence band of the crystal. Electrons are raised to the conduction band, where they roam free. The vacancy left in the valence band is known as an *electron-hole*. The vacancy is soon filled by another electron from the same band, and this process repeats itself many times. The result is that, while electrons travel free in the conduction band, electron-holes travel free in the valence band. Soon, electrons in the conduction band fall into electron traps in the forbidden band, and holes rise to hole traps in the same band. Upon heating in a special instrument, electrons and holes in the forbidden band recombine, releasing energy in the form of visible light.

The intensity of the light released is measured with a photomultiplier tube (PMT) in a similar fashion as scintillations are measured in gamma cameras or other scintillation detectors.

3. Quantification

LiF crystals are embedded into soft tissue equivalent plastic to make the so-called TLD chips. This design permits reading of doses directly in millirems or μSv. A calibration curve is prepared by exposing TLD chips to various known doses from an NBS-certified source of gamma rays or a well-calibrated x-ray machine. The chips are then heated and read using a special instrument. The readings are expressed

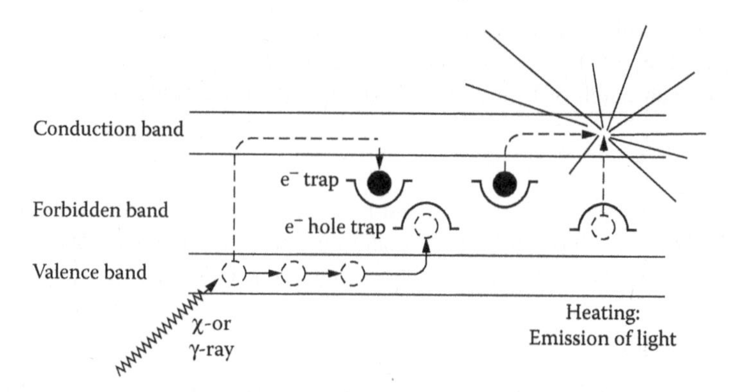

FIGURE 8.5 Diagram of a TLD crystal. Exposure to radiation causes electrons and electron holes to fall into traps in the forbidden band. Upon heating, they recombine, releasing light of intensity proportional to absorbed radiation dose.

in terms of "counts." A computer plots counts vs. doses. The data on the curve can now be used to convert readings from TLD badges and TLD rings, worn by radiation workers, into doses.

4. The Service

TLD service is available commercially. Hospitals and clinics can contract the service with a certified provider. Radiation workers can be monitored for whole-body exposure with TLD badges and for hand exposure with TLD ring dosimeters. Figure 8.6 shows a TLD badge, its design, identification of the wearer, and the TLD chips set behind calibration filters. Badges are to be worn on the laboratory coat at a level closest to the sources handled. Figure 8.7 shows a TLD ring dosimeter, its design, and the choice of three ring sizes. Ring dosimeters are recommended for radiopharmacists, NMTs, and students of NMT in training. TLD rings are to be worn with the chip facing the palm of the preferred hand.

5. Advantages of TLD

TLD dosimeters are more sensitive than films. They can reliably record exposures down to 1 mrem (10 μSv). Readings are given directly in mrem or μSv. TLDs are not significantly affected by weather conditions and are reusable.

6. Disadvantages of TLD

TLD service is more expensive than that of film dosimetry. Once read, the information is lost. Calibration curves must be prepared with each batch.

D. Pocket Dosimeters

1. Description

Pocket dosimeters are ionization chambers designed to be worn like a pocket pen. They operate as an electroscope. Cumulative doses can be read at any time during

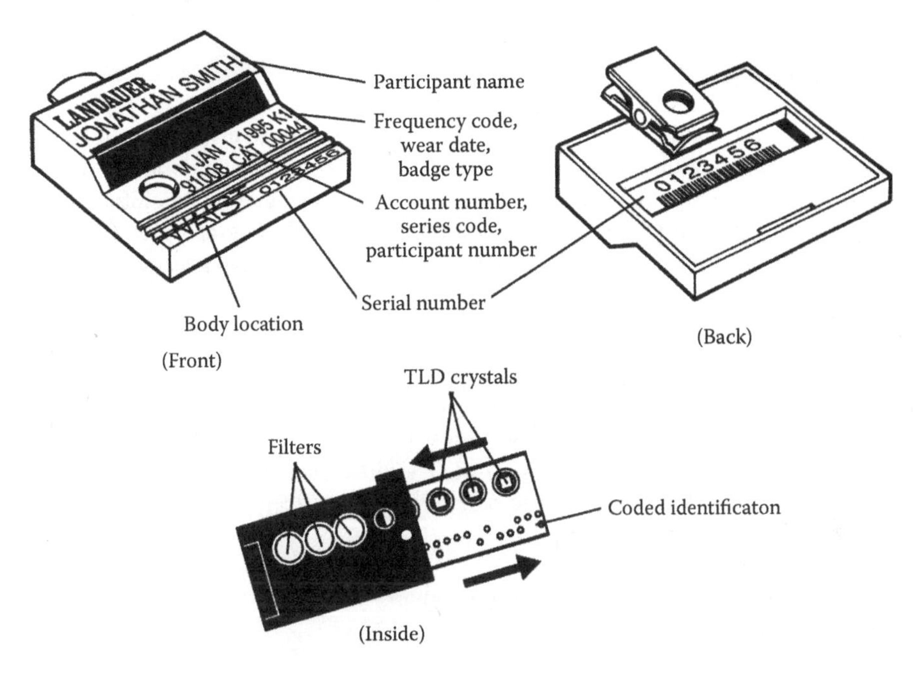

FIGURE 8.6 TLD badge. The case design, the method of identification, and the TLD crystal holder are shown. (Courtesy of Landauer, Inc., Glenwood, IL.)

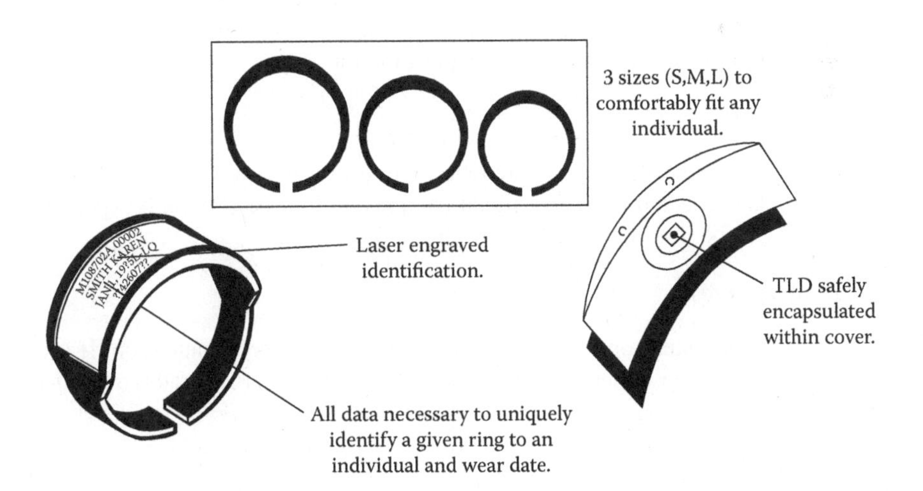

FIGURE 8.7 TLD ring dosimeter. A choice of three sizes and the identification method are shown. (Courtesy of Landauer, Inc., Gleenwood, IL.)

work. Their design and operation was described in Chapter 4. A diagram is shown in Figure 4.3. Reference was made to them also in Chapter 5.

2. Advantages

Pocket dosimeters are sensitive instruments. They can provide instant dose readings when performing certain operations such as drawing a therapeutic dose of ^{131}I from a multidose vial. Worn on the collar, chest pocket, or waist, they can monitor whole-body exposure; worn on the wrist of the preferred hand, they can measure hand dose; and when worn inside a lead apron, a pregnant worker can measure fetal dose.

3. Disadvantages

Pocket dosimeters are fragile. When dropped accidentally, the information is lost. When recharged, the previous information is lost. Reliable daily readings and recordings are required. Each day, the wearer must perform two readings: upon entering the working areas and upon leaving work. The difference between the readings is the dose received during the day. The radiation safety officer (RSO) must verify the records daily.

E. Personal Alarm Monitors (Bleepers)

1. Description

Personal alarm monitors are small GM detectors contained in a box about 10- to 12-cm long, 7.5-cm wide, and 2.5-cm deep. They weigh about 120 to 160 g. They can be worn on the laboratory coat pocket or on the belt. They provide visual readout of cumulative dose or dose rate as well as an audible signal. They can also show cumulative dose up to 1000 mrem (10 mSv). A small ^{137}Cs source is used to verify proper operation. Figure 5.6 shows a bleeper monitor.

2. Advantages

Personal alarm monitors (blippers) are extremely useful in a very active radiopharmacy or hot lab. The audible alarm signal can prevent unnecessary high exposures. This device can be used in addition to a film or TLD badge.

3. Disadvantages

Because they are battery operated, these monitors require special attention. If used as the only monitoring method, readings must be reliably and accurately recorded.

F. OSL Dosimetry

OSL stands for optically stimulated luminescence, a method of dosimetry that uses aluminum oxide (Al_2O_3) crystals activated with traces of carbon. After exposure, the crystals are stimulated by a laser that induces luminescence. Immediately, the luminescence is read with a PMT. The intensity of luminescence is proportional to the radiation dose received.

1. Advantages

OSL dosimeters are more sensitive than TLDs. They can be read and reused several times.

2. Disadvantages

Because of their low Z number, they are not tissue equivalent.

V. RECORDS OF PERSONNEL DOSIMETRY

A. Personnel Doses

Each licensee must keep records of the annual dose received by all radiation workers, which includes the whole-body deep equivalent dose, the whole-body and extremity shallow equivalent dose, and the lens equivalent dose (10CFR20.2106). These records are to be kept on NRC Form 5 or its equivalent. Monthly service providers' reports are equivalent.

B. Previous Records

An attempt to obtain the personal radiation exposure history (cumulative dose) of each worker must be made by the licensee. This includes obtaining the exposure history from previous employment. These data are recorded on NRC Form 4 or its equivalent. If a record of the previous dose is not available, the dose limits will be assumed as received in order to arrive at the best estimate of the worker's cumulative dose (10CFR20.2104).

C. Committed Dose

If required, the licensee must keep records of the annual committed effective equivalent dose for each worker. This record must be entered on NRC Form 5 or its equivalent.

D. Other Records

1. If needed, fetal dose must be recorded for all declared pregnancies.
2. If required, records of radiation monitoring of nonrestricted areas must also be kept.
3. All personnel dose records are to be kept for the duration of the license.

VI. REPORTS

A. Lost or Stolen Radioactive Sources

Regulations require that a telephone report be made to the licensing agency immediately after the discovery of a missing radioactive source. This is followed by a written report within 30 d of the loss if the source has not been recovered by then. The report must include measures taken to prevent future similar events (10CFR20.2201).

B. Incident Reports (10CFR20.2202)

According to regulations, all personnel exceeding occupational dose limits must be reported to the licensing agency as follows:

1. Immediate Notification

a. Required for all whole-body doses exceeding 25 rem (250 mSv).
b. Lens dose exceeding 75 rem (750 mSv).
c. Hand doses exceeding 250 rem (2.5 Sv).
d. Immediate notification is also required for any radioactivity releases that would result in five times the annual limits on intake (5 × ALI).

2. Twenty-Four-Hour Notification

Required for all whole-body doses, eye lens doses, and hand doses exceeding the annual occupational dose limits, as well as any radioactivity releases that would result in one ALI.

VII. REPORTABLE EVENTS

A. Incidents

Regulations mandate that written reports to the licensing agencies must be made within 30 d of the incidents or source losses mentioned earlier. Such reports must contain a description of corrective measures to prevent future similar incidents.

B. The EPA

Licensees subject to EPA regulations must report radioactivity releases exceeding EPA standards.

C. Reports to Individuals

Individuals who exceed 10% of the annual dose limits (whole-body dose, organ dose, lens dose, shallow dose, extremity dose, or ALI) must be notified of their annual dose received on NRC Form 5 or its equivalent. A signed copy must be kept on file by the licensee.

D. Files

Copies of all reports are to be kept on file for the duration of the license (CFR20.2005).

PROBLEMS

Questions in this chapter concern radionuclide generators and their eluants. Please refer to Chapter 1 and Chapter 5 for assistance.

1. A ^{99m}Tc generator arrives Monday at 8:00 a.m. containing 24 GBq of ^{99}Mo. What will its activity be at 11:00 a.m. on Friday?
2. An eluant contains 13 GBq of ^{99m}Tc in 10 ml at 8:00 a.m. What will its concentration be at 11:00 a.m.?
3. What category of shipping packages are ^{99m}Tc generators, and what is the dose rate limit on their surfaces at shipping time?
4. The concentration of a ^{99m}Tc eluant is 2.4 GBq/ml at 8:00 a.m. What volume will contain 4.0 GBq at 10:30 a.m.?
5. A ^{99m}Tc generator is shipped at noon on Friday containing 28 GBq of ^{99}Mo. What will its activity be at 8:00 a.m. on Monday?
6. A ^{99m}Tc eluant contains 0.10 μCi of ^{99}Mo per millicurie of ^{99m}Tc at 8:00 a.m. At what time will the eluant reach the limit of 0.15?
7. A ^{99m}Tc eluant contains 50 nCi of ^{99}Mo per millicurie of ^{99m}Tc at 8:00 a.m. Can the eluant be used within the next eight working hours?
8. An eluant of ^{99m}Tc has a concentration of 2.0 GBq/ml at 9:00 a.m. What volume will contain 3.0 GBq/ml at 4:00 p.m.?
9. The concentration of a ^{99m}Tc eluant is 1.5 GBq/ml at 8:00 p.m. What volume must be drawn at 11:00 a.m. for a dosage of 740 MBq?
10. A ^{99m}Tc generator contains 1.18 GBq of ^{99}Mo on Wednesday at noon. What was the activity on the previous Monday at 8:00 a.m.?

REFERENCES

Bernier, D.R., Christian, P.E., and Langan, J.K., *Nuclear Medicine Technology and Techniques*, 3d ed., Mosby, St. Louis, 1994.

Bevalacqua, J.J., *Basic Health Physics — Problems and Solutions*, Wiley–VCH, Weinheim, Germany, 1999.

Code of Federal Regulations, Title 10, National Archives Records Administration, Washington, DC, 2005.

Chandra, R., *Nuclear Medicine Physics — The Basics*, 6th ed., Lippincott Williams & Wilkins, Philadelphia, 2004.

Dowd, S.B. and Tilson, E.R., *Practical Radiation Protection and Applied Radiobiology*, 2d ed., Saunders, 1999.

Early, P.J., *Review of Rules and Regulations Governing the Practice of Nuclear Medicine*, 41st Annual Meeting of the Society of Nuclear Medicine, Orlando, 1994.

Early, P.J. and Sodee, D.B., *Principles and Practice of Nuclear Medicine*, 2d ed., Mosby, St. Louis, 1995.

Klingensmith, W.C., Eshima, D., and Goddard, J., *Nuclear Medicine Procedure Manual*, Oxford Medical, Englewood, NJ, 1991.

Kowalsky, R.J. and Falen, S.W., *Radiopharmaceuticals in Nuclear Pharmacy and Nuclear Medicine*, 2d ed., American Pharmacists Association, Washington, DC, 2004.

Man–Sung, Y., *A Guide to Personnel Monitoring for Radiation in the Hospital Environment*, Landauer, Glenwood, IL, 1993.

Mason, J.S., Elliott, K.M., and Mitro, A.C., *The Nuclear Medicine Handbook for Achieving Compliance with NRC Regulations*, Society of Nuclear Medicine, Reston, VA, 1997.

Noz, M.E. and Maguire, G.Q., *Radiation Protection in the Radiological and Health Sciences*, 2d ed., Lea and Febiger, Philadelphia, 1995.

Saha, G.B., *Physics of Radiobiology and Nuclear Medicine*, Springer–Verlag, New York, 1993.

Sandler, M.P. et al., Editors, (Coleman, Patton, Wackers, and Gottschalk), *Diagnostic Nuclear Medicine*, Lippincott Williams & Wilkins, Philadelphia, 2003.

Silverstein, E.B. et al., *Society of Nuclear Medicine Procedure Guideline for Palliative Treatment of Painful Bone Metastases*, Society of Nuclear Medicine, Reston, VA, 2003.

Statkiewicz-Sherer, M.A., Visconti, P.J., and Ritenour, E.R., *Radiation Protection in Medical Radiography*, 2d ed., Mosby, St. Louis, 1993.

Steves, A.M., *Review of Nuclear Medicine Technology*, 2d ed., Society of Nuclear Medicine, Reston, VA, 1996.

Zimmerman, R.L., *Important Information about Radiation Monitoring Badges and Records*, Nexus, Landauer, Glenwood, IL, 1993.

9 Internal Dosimetry and Bioassays

I. RATIONALE

The RSO receives the monthly report of film and TLD dosimetry with expectation and concern. Expectation, because he/she expects that none of the staff had received a radiation dose greater than 10% of the dose limits in accordance with ALARA. And concern, because if someone received a dose exceeding the 10% level or the 30% level, he/she must interview the person to determine the cause and possibly avoid such events in the future.

In NM, most radiation doses are due to external exposures. Internal doses are avoided by heeding some basic laboratory rules, by proper handling, and by following the procedure protocols exactly. However, as the number of PET imaging and radionuclide therapy procedures continues to expand, radiation workers must remain more vigilant and apply stricter rules to prevent internal contamination by accidental ingestion, inhalation, or percutaneous absorption.

Regarding patients, it is very reassuring to know that most imaging procedures deliver very low internal doses and that, in these cases, the benefits clearly outweigh the risks of very low radiation doses. Patients under radionuclide therapy, on the other hand, receive large radiation doses to target malignant tissues. But they benefit too because the treatment is aimed at stopping and possibly curing them from their illness.

The objectives of this chapter are (a) to present a historical review of internal dosimetry, (b) to provide the readers with a best estimate of internal dosimetry from radiopharmaceuticals, and (c) to explain the basics of bioassays following the accidental intake of radioactivity.

II. HISTORICAL REVIEW

A. General Considerations

The effective equivalent dose and the internal organ equivalent dose are the result of several factors:

1. The quantity of radioactivity in the body
2. The types, abundance, and energies of the radiation emissions
3. The size, weight, and shape of organs and the whole body
4. The rates of organ uptake and organ excretion

5. The retention times in some organs and in the whole body
6. The fractional energy absorbed within those organs and the whole body

B. Methods

From the historical point of view, two methods are described:

1. The ICRP method, based strictly on the physical properties of radiations.
2. The MIRD (medical internal radiation dose) method, which uses a more realistic mathematical approach to uptake, retention, and absorbed radiation energies.

Also described is RADAR (radiation dose assessment resource), a web site that is provided to the medical community by an international team of experts.

C. The ICRP Method

The ICRP proposed a method based on the amount of radioactivity taken up by the organ, the mass of the organ, and the retention time within the organ.

1. Assumptions

a. Most organs are like spheres. They have an "effective radius."
b. Organ uptakes are instantaneous, and the radioactivity is uniformly distributed throughout the organ.
c. Patients resemble "standard man," (70-kg weight, 1.70-m tall).
d. Patients should tolerate occupational dose limits.

Although the ICRP assumptions are not valid today, they were considered reasonable when they were proposed even though they overestimated internal doses. The methods are based on Marinelli's equations given in the following text.

2. "Standard Man"

In 1975, the ICRP defined what, at the time, represented the average man in the United States: A man, 20 to 30 y of age, weighing 70 kg (154 lb), 1.70 m tall (5 ft, 7 in.), living in a climate whose temperature oscillated between 10 and 30°C (50 and 86°F). During the years that followed, some adjustments were made to arrive at a better definition of the average man. Table 9.1 gives the masses of some internal organs of a standard man.

3. The Snyder–Fisher Phantom

Under the sponsorship of the U.S. Department of Energy, the Snyder–Fisher phantom was built to correspond to the exact body size and weight, organ sizes, weights, and densities of standard man. Using films and TLD chips, implanted in the phantom, as well as radioactive solutions filling the internal organs, the phantom was used to confirm or correct internal dosimetry calculations. In later years, other phantoms

TABLE 9.1
Some Organ Masses of Standard Man

Organ	Mass (kg)	Organ	Mass (kg)
Muscle	28	Large intestine	0.37
Skeleton	5.12	Kidneys	0.31
Skin	2.6	Spleen	0.18
Liver	1.8	Stomach wall	0.15
Red marrow	1.5	Bladder wall	0.045
Lungs	1.0	Thyroid gland	0.020
Small intestine	0.64	Whole body	70.0

were designed for women, pregnant women in various stages of gestation, and children of various ages.

3. The Marinelli Equations

Beta and gamma doses use two different equations:

(a) Beta dose equation:

$$D_\beta = 73.8C\bar{E}_\beta T_e \quad (9.1)$$

where D_β = beta dose in rads, 73.8 = constant resulting from conversion of units, C = concentration in μCi/g, $\bar{E}_\beta$ = average energy of beta particles, in MeV, and T_e = effective half-life, in days.

(b) Gamma dose equation:

$$D_\gamma = 0.0346\ C\Gamma g T_e \quad (9.2)$$

where D_γ = gamma dose in rads, 0.0346 = constant resulting from conversion of units, C = concentration in μCi/g, Γ = specific gamma constant in R/mCi-h at 1 cm, g = geometry factor = $3\pi r$, assuming a sphere of radius r, and T_e = effective half-time in days.

4. Effective Half-Life (T_e)

Effective half-life, or effective half-time, is the time in which half of the radioactivity is removed from the organ or from the whole body by the combined processes of radioactive decay and biological excretion. If biological excretion is a single exponential function of time, then the following applies:

$$T_e = (T_p \times T_b)/(T_p + T_b) \quad (9.3)$$

where T_p = physical (radioactive) half-life and T_b = biological half-life.

Sample Problems

(a) What is the whole-body beta dose from 1 mCi of tritiated water given to a 70-kg person assuming an effective half-time of 12 d?
Solution: $D_\beta = 73.8\ (1000\ \mu Ci/70{,}000\ g)\ 0.006\ MeV \times 12\ d = 0.076\ rad$

(b) What is the gamma dose to the liver of a 60-kg patient assuming a 2-mCi uptake of ^{99m}Tc-S-colloid in a spherical liver and indefinite retention?
Solution:
Liver mass = 1800 g × 60 kg/70 kg = 1642 g
Concentration = 2000 μCi/1642 g = 1.3 μCi/g
^{99m}Tc specific gamma constant = 0.78 R/mCi h at 1 cm
Geometric factor, 1642-g sphere = 67.55
Effective half-life: 6 h = 0.25 d
$D_\gamma = 0.0346 \times 1.3\ \mu Ci/g \times 0.78\ R/mCi\text{-}h \times 67.55 \times 0.25\ d = 0.592\ rad$

D. The MIRD Method

In the 1960s, the Society of Nuclear Medicine (SNM) formed the Medical Internal Radiation Dose (MIRD) Committee with the charge of designing an accurate method for calculating internal doses from diagnostic and therapeutic doses of radiopharmaceuticals. The results of its work were published in several supplements of the *Journal of Nuclear Medicine* (JNM) in the years that followed. The Society's method is believed to be more accurate than that of the ICRP. A brief description is given here.

1. MIRD Assumptions

a. Internal organs are not spheres. They are more like ellipsoids, cyllindroids, conical cyllindroids, or prolate cyllindroids.
b. Uptake by organs is not instantaneous. It is more like an exponential function of time (Figure 9.1).
c. Organ retention times are variable. Concentration is homogeneous.
d. Removal from the organ can be represented by a single or a composite exponential function of time (Figure 9.1).

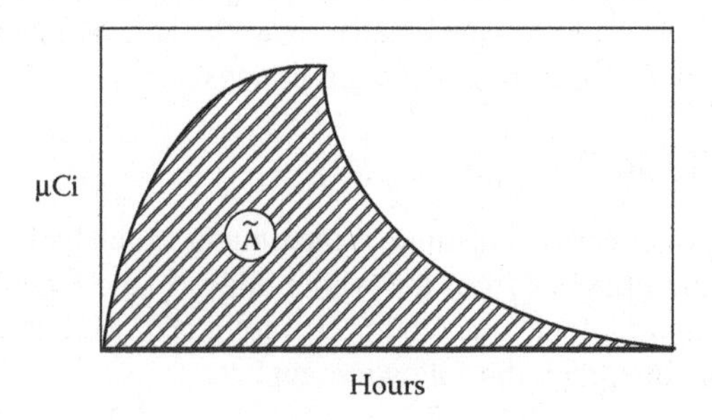

FIGURE 9.1 Cumulative activity (Ã) is the residence time of the radioactivity in an organ. In the figure, Ã is represented by the shaded area under the curve. Ã is expressed in μCi-h.

TABLE 9.2
Some Equilibrium Dose Constants

Radionuclide	(g-rad/μCi h)
Fluorine-18	2.6272
Phosphorus-32	1.4799
Iodine-131	1.2131
Indium-111	0.9421
Gallium-67	0.4169
Iodine-123	0.4202
Xenon-133	0.3878
Technetium-99m	0.3029
Iodine-125	0.1347

e. The area under the curve in Figure 9.1 represents the cumulative activity ($\tilde{A}$) or residence time and is expressed in μCi-h.
f. In addition to standard man, standard woman, and standard children of various ages are to be considered.
g. For each subject, basic biological (kinetic) data must be obtained to arrive at more accurate residence times.

2. The MIRD Equations

$$D = (\tilde{A}/m)\Sigma\Delta_i\phi_i \tag{9.4}$$

where D = dose in rad, $\tilde{A}$ = cumulative activity, m = organ mass in grams, Σ = sum of, Δ_i = equilibrium dose constant in g rad/μCi-h, and ϕ_i = absorbed fraction, from MIRD tables.

3. Cumulative Activities ($\tilde{A}$)

Cumulative activities are the product of the activity (A) in microcuries times the mean effective half-life in hours:

$$\tilde{A} = A1.443T_e \tag{9.5}$$

4. Equilibrium Dose Constants (Δ_i)

For each radiation emission (beta, gamma, conversion electrons, x-rays, and Auger electrons), Δ_i is the product of their abundances (n_i) times their mean energies (E_i) and the sum of all the products. MIRD tabulated these for many radionuclides of medical interest. Table 9.2 shows some examples.

5. Absorbed Fraction (ϕ_i)

Absorbed fraction is the ratio of the energy absorbed by the organ to the energy emitted by the source. For nonpenetrating radiations — particles and photons of less

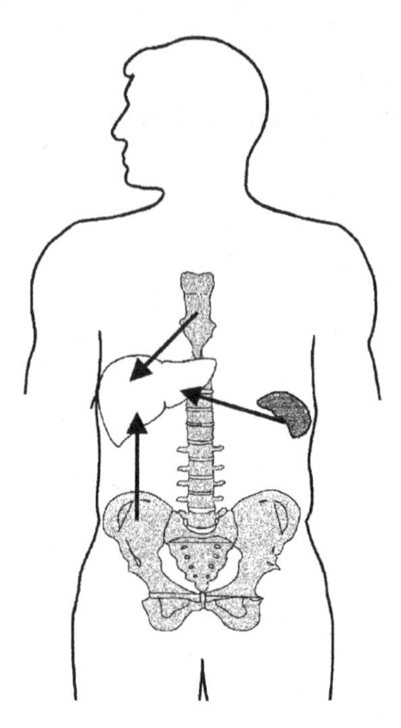

FIGURE 9.2 Radiation dose to the liver after the administration of ^{99m}Tc-S-colloid. Diagramatically, the liver receives radiation from itself (liver-to-liver dose), from the spleen (spleen-to-liver dose), and from the bone marrow (bone-marrow-to-liver dose).

than 11 keV — the absorbed fractions are equal to one (complete absorption). For penetrating radiations — x-rays and gamma rays >11 keV — absorbed fractions have been calculated and measured using Monte Carlo technique algorithms and the standard man phantom. The Monte Carlo technique calculates the probabilities of interactions of each type of radiation within an organ or within the whole body. MIRD has tabulated these and published them in the JNM, supplements 3 and 8.

6. Effective Absorbed Energies (EAE)

In an attempt to simplify calculations, the MIRD Committee multiplied, for each radiation emission, the equilibrium dose constants times their absorbed fractions and then added the products. The results were the EAEs, which were also published in the form of tables for many situations, such as target-to-target-organ, source-organ-to-target-organ, etc. For example, Figure 9.2 shows that from ^{99m}Tc-S-colloid, the liver receives radiation doses from itself, the spleen, and the bone marrow. According to MIRD, the target organ dose then becomes

$$D = (\tilde{A}/m)\ EAE \tag{9.6}$$

7. Mean Absorbed Doses (S)

In another attempt to simplify calculations, the MIRD Committee introduced the "S values," or mean absorbed dose/unit of cumulative activity, which is nothing

TABLE 9.3
Reported Dosimetries

Radiopharmaceutical	Organ	(rad/mCi)	(μSv/MBq)
^{99m}Tc-RBC	Spleen	0.11	30
^{99m}Tc-pertechnetate	ULI	0.12	32
	Thyroid	0.13	35
^{99m}Tc-MDP	Bladder[a]	0.13	35
^{99m}Tc-pyrophosphate	Bone surfaces	0.14	38
^{99m}Tc-depreotide	Spleen	0.16	42
	Kidneys	0.33	90
^{99m}Tc-sestamibi	ULI[a]	0.18	49
^{99m}Tc-apcitide	Bladder	0.22	60
^{99m}Tc-MAA	Lungs	0.22	59
^{99m}Tc-lanolesomab	Spleen	0.24	64
^{99m}Tc-DMSA	Renal cortex	0.85	230
^{99m}Tc-S-colloid	Liver	0.34	91.8
^{123}I-iofetamine	Bladder	0.23	62
^{67}Ga-citrate	Spleen	0.53	143
	ULI	0.56	151
	Bone marrow	0.58	157
	LLI	0.90	243
^{123}I-MIBG	Adrenal medulla	0.80	216
^{111}In-pentetreotide	Spleen	2.46	664

[a] 2-h void.

other than the EAEs divided by the organ weights of standard man. The absorbed dose is then

$$D = \tilde{A} \times S \tag{9.7}$$

The MIRD Committee has also published S-value tables so that NM professionals could use them in their internal dosimetry calculations. But simplification has its price. The S values are accurate for standard man, but very few persons are like standard man.

8. Internal Doses According to MIRD

Internal organs that receive the highest radiation doses from diagnostic RPs are referred to as *critical organs*. Table 9.3 shows the doses received by critical organs in terms of rad/mCi and μSv/MBq. The data shown were obtained using MIRD tables and equations.

E. The RADAR Web Site

In 2002, a group of international experts started RADAR (radiation dose assessment resource), a web site dedicated to provide dosimetry services to the medical community. The site address is www.doseinfo-radar.com. Visitors can enter a number of combinations of radiologic and NM procedures and the amounts of radioactivities used. The answers are given for internal organ doses and total effective doses in mrems and in mSv. Physicians can use these answers prospectively, to plan an NM procedure, or retrospectively, to research case studies on their files.

III. INTERNAL DOSES FROM RADIOPHARMACEUTICALS

A. Package Inserts

1. Requirement

As required by the FDA, radiopharmaceutical companies must provide the medical community with basic important information about the safety and efficacy of their products. Among the safety information is the radiodosimetry of internal organ doses and total effective doses. Some of that data is presented in tabulated form in the following sections.

B. Diagnostic RPs

1. Conventional Imaging Procedures

Table 9.3 contains data reported by many RP manufacturers, adapted and presented in the two systems of units. With very few exceptions, the doses to critical organs (those receiving the highest doses) are well below one rad per millicurie. That is expected in diagnostic NM.

2. Dosimetry of ^{18}F-FDG

Organs such as the brain and the myocardium have a relatively high metabolic rate, and consequently, they take up a high fraction of the dosage of ^{18}F-FDG. Similarly, malignant tumors also have a high metabolic rate, and therefore, they glow under the PET scanner. The diagnostic value of PET represents a quantum leap in the practice of medicine. In recent times, the number of PET procedures has increased very fast, and this trend is expected to continue in the near future. Table 9.4 shows the radiation doses received by critical organs of patients subjected to PET imaging with ^{18}F-FDG. Doses are similar to those shown in Table 9.3.

3. Dosimetry of Radionuclide Therapy

As described in Chapter 6, pure negatron emitters such as ^{32}P, ^{89}Sr, ^{90}Sr, ^{153}Sm, ^{90}Y, ^{186}Re, ^{188}Re, and ^{177}Lu, are prescribed to treat malignant illnesses or to palliate the pain of bone metastases. ^{32}P-colloidal suspensions are used in intracavitary therapy. Murine and humanized monoclonal antibodies labelled with ^{90}Y or ^{131}I are prescribed in the treatment of malignant lymphomas. Table 9.5 lists the dosimetries of ^{131}I iodide; Table 9.6 gives the dosimetry of agents used in the palliation of pain in

TABLE 9.4
Dosimetry of ^{18}F-FDG

Organ	(rad/mCi)	(μSv/MBq)
Spleen	0.044	12
Kidneys	0.078	21
Brain	0.096	26
Bladder, 1-h void	0.220	59
Bladder, 2-h void	0.440	119
Bladder	0.629	170
Heart	0.241	65
Whole body	0.043	12
Fetus (3 months)	0.081	22

TABLE 9.5
Dosimetry of ^{131}I Therapy

Therapy Level	Organ	(rad/mCi)	(mSv/MBq)
^{131}I-Iodide (10-mCi level)	Thyroid	13,000	3,510
	Stomach	14	3.78
	Ovaries	1.4	0.378
^{131}I-Iodide (29-mCi level)	Thyroid	37,700	10,200
	Stomach	40.6	11
	Ovaries	4.1	1.11
	Testes	2.6	0.7
^{131}I-Iodide (150 mCi level)	Thyroid	39,000	10,500
	Stomach	255	68.9
	Liver	30	8.1
	Marrow	21	5.67
	Ovaries	21	5.67

TABLE 9.6
Palliation of Pain in Bone Metastases

Therapeutic Agent	Organ	(rad/mCi)	(mSv/MBq)
^{32}P-phosphate	Bone surface	37.0	10
	Red bone marrow	28.1	7.6
^{89}Sr-chloride	Bone surface	63.0	17.0
	Red bone marrow	40.7	11.0
	LLI	17.4	4.7
	Bladder	4.8	1.3
	Kidneys	3.0	0.8
^{153}Sm-EDTMP	Bone surface	25.0	6.8
	Red bone marrow	5.7	1.5
	Bladder wall	3.6	1.0

TABLE 9.7
Dosimetry of Therapy with Monoclonal Antibodies

Therapeutic Agent	Organ	(rad/mCi)	(mSv/MBq)
^{131}I-Tositumomab	Thyroid	10.0	2.71
	Kidneys	7.3	1.96
	ULI	5.0	1.34
	LLI	4.6	1.30
	Spleen	4.2	1.14
^{125}I-B72.3 MAb	Thyroid	7.90	2.13
	Bladder	0.54	0.15
^{90}Y-Ibritumomab	Spleen	34.8	9.4
Tiuxetan	Testes	33.7	9.1
	Liver	17.8	4.8
	LLI	17.8	4.8
	ULI	13.3	3.6
	Heart	10.4	2.8
	Lungs	7.4	2.0
	SI	5.2	1.4
	Marrow	4.8	1.3

patients with bone metastases; and Table 9.7 shows the dosimetry of some radiolabelled monoclonal antibodies used in the therapy of malignant illnesses.

4. Diagnostic Whole-Body and Fetal Doses

In general, diagnostic whole-body doses are extremely low. For a given RP, they vary between 1 and 10% of the doses to critical organs. When ^{99m}Tc or ^{123}I imaging procedures are prescribed to pregnant patients, it is very reassuring to know that fetal doses are even lower.

IV. BIOASSAY OF RADIOACTIVITY

A. Definitions

Radiobioassays are laboratory tests that quantify the accidental intake of radioactivity in the body of radiation workers. The method of assay can be direct, using a whole-body counter, or indirect, by calculation from analyses of samples obtained from the contaminated workers. Analytical procedures must be simple, rapid, sensitive, accurate, and inexpensive.

1. Intake: Quantity of a radionuclide entering the body by inhalation, ingestion, or through the skin (percutaneous absorption or accidental injection)
2. Uptake: Quantity of a radionuclide transferred from the site of intake to other organs or tissues

TABLE 9.8
Occupational ALIs and DACs in Nuclear Medicine

Nuclide	ALI, Ingestion (μCi)	ALI, Inhalation (μCi)	DAC, Inhalation (μCi/ml)
^{99m}Tc	8×10^4	2×10^5	1×10^{-4}
^{18}F	5×10^4	7×10^4	3×10^{-5}
^{125}I	4×10^1	6×10^1	3×10^{-6}
^{32}P	6×10^3	3×10^3	1×10^{-6}
^{131}I	9×10^1	5×10^1	2×10^{-8}

3. Retained quantity: Quantity of a radionuclide in a tissue or organ at some time after the intake or uptake
4. Urinary excretion: Removal of radioactivity from the body by the urinary system
5. Fecal excretion: Removal of endogenous or exogenous radioactivity by the GI tract

B. Requirements

Regulations require that each licensee monitor the occupational intake of radioactivity and assess the committed effective dose to any worker likely to receive more than 10% of the ALI (annual limit on intake). In certain cases, continuous monitoring of the NM department for DACs (derived air concentrations) may be required.

C. Airborne Medical Radionuclides

Table 9.8 shows the occupational limits for ALIs by ingestion and inhalation and DACs by inhalation of NM radionuclides with some potential for being airborne. Exceeding those limits would result in a total effective equivalent dose greater than 5 rem/y and internal organ equivalent dose greater than 50 rem/y.

D. Bioassays of Iodine-131

Regulations require that each licensee monitor the thyroid burden of workers involved in the preparation and administration of therapeutic quantities of ^{131}I to patients. This can be done by the thyroid uptake test, using suitable standards, at 24, 48, and 72 h. Indirectly, the thyroid burden can also be determined by an accurate assay of quantitative urine samples.

1. Alert and Action Levels for ^{131}I

a. Alert level I (Evaluation): 2% of ALI (2% of 50 μCi), determined as follows:

$$50\ \mu\text{Ci} \times 0.02 \times 0.133 = 0.133\ \mu\text{Ci}\ (4.92\ \text{kBq})$$

where 0.133 is the retention factor.

b. Alert level II (Investigational): 10% of ALI:

$$50\ \mu\text{Ci} \times 0.10 \times 0.133 = 0.633\ \mu\text{Ci}\ (23.42\ \text{kBq})$$

2. Action Levels

More than 2% of ALI: Repeat bioassays
More than 10% of ALI: Repeat bioassays, institute air sampling, strict surveys
More than 3 μCi (111 kBq): Consider stopping use of ^{131}I
More than 6 μCi (222 kBq): Stop using ^{131}I

E. Biological Models

Two metabolic models are of interest.

1. Highly Diffusible Radionuclides

These are radionuclides that disperse quickly throughout the whole body. Within minutes, the body behaves as a single compartment. Immediately after that, the radionuclide leaves the body as a single exponential function of time. Examples of such radionuclides are ^{3}H (tritium), ^{22}Na, ^{24}Na, ^{36}Cl, and ^{137}Cs. Figure 9.3 shows the whole-body compartment and the radionuclide removal curve. The general equation is

$$\text{Percentage remaining} = 100e^{-\lambda_b t} \tag{9.8}$$

where e = base of natural logarithms (2.71828...), λ_b = biological constant = ln $2/T_b$, T_b = biological half-time, and t = elapsed time.

The fraction of the initial body burden present in the sample is called the excretion function $E_{(t)}$. The equation is

$$E_{(t)} = (\ln 2 / T_b)e^{-\lambda_b t} \tag{9.9}$$

Sample Problem

A 68-kg radiochemist was exposed to an accidental intake of T_2O (tritiated water). A 24-h urine sample (1,450 ml) taken on the third day, measured with a liquid scintillation counter whose efficiency was 40%, yielded 6,750 net c/min/ml. Assuming a T_b = 10 d, calculate (a) the percent remaining in the body, (b) the activity in the sample, (c) the excretion function, and (d) the initial body burden.

Solution:

a. Percentage remaining (Equation 9.8): (answer: 93.3%).
b. Activity in sample: $(6{,}752 \times 1{,}450)/(0.4 \times 2.22 \times 10^6) = 11$ μCi (408 kBq).
c. Excretion function (Equation 9.9): (answer: 6.46% in sample).
d. Initial body burden = 11 μCi/0.0646 = 165.7 μCi (6.31 MBq).

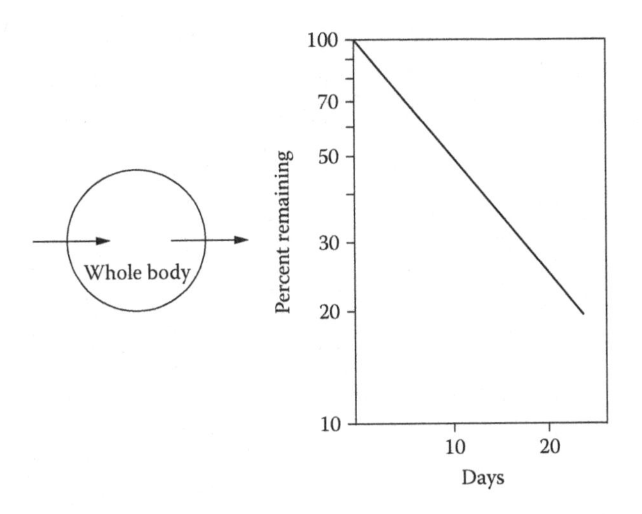

FIGURE 9.3 Model for a highly diffusible radionuclide. The whole body behaves as a single compartment at a steady state. The remaining radioactivity is a single exponential function of time.

2. High-Organ-Uptake Radionuclides

These are radionuclides that are taken up and retained by one or more internal organs. For example, all radioiodines, especially ^{131}I and ^{125}I, are taken and retained by the thyroid gland. Other organs may take significant amounts of radioiodine, but their retention times are very short. Those organs are the gastric mucosa, the salivary glands, the choroid plexus of the brain, the kidneys, and the bladder. The model is represented by a composite of exponentials, which can be reduced to two components: a slow component, represented by the thyroid gland, and a fast component, represented by the other organs and the whole body. Figure 9.4 shows the body and the high-uptake organ on the left, and the composite exponential removal curve on the right. The equation for that curve is the following:

$$\text{Percentage remaining} = Ae^{-\lambda_{b1}t} + Be^{-\lambda_{b2}t} \tag{9.10}$$

where A = fast component y-intercept, B = slow component y-intercept, λ_{b1} = excretion rate, fast component, λ_{b2} = excretion rate, slow component, and t = elapsed time.

The excretion function for radioiodine, assuming $T_1 = 0.35$ d and $T_2 = 100$ d is

$$E_{(t)} = [4.37e^{-1.98t} + 0.002e^{-0.007t}]e^{-0.0861t} \tag{9.11}$$

Sample Problem

A technician was accidentally exposed to ^{131}I. A 24-h sample of urine (1660 ml), taken on the second day after exposure, yielded 75 net c/min/ml in a well-type scintillation counter. A 0.1-μCi standard of ^{131}I yielded 7250 c/min. Calculate the initial body burden.

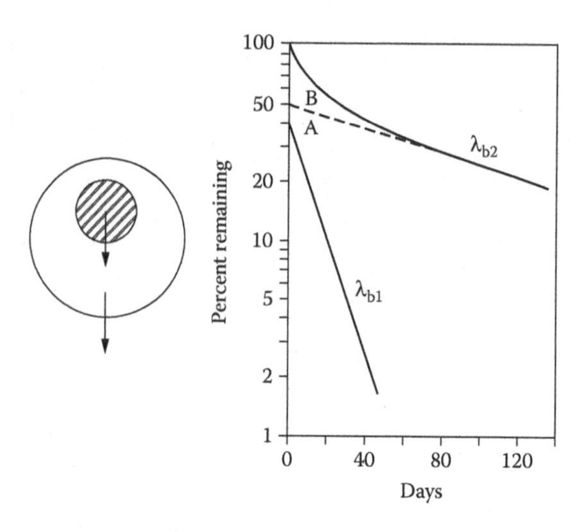

FIGURE 9.4 Model for a high-organ-uptake radionuclide. The whole-body remaining radioactivity is a composite exponential function of time. A and B are the y-intercepts of the fast and slow components, respectively; λ_{b1} and λ_{b2} are fast and slow removal rates (slopes), respectively.

Solution:

a. Activity in the sample: (75 × 0.1/7250) 1,660 = 1.72 μCi (second day)
b. Excretion function (Equation 9.11): (answer: 7.18 % of initial burden)
c. Initial body burden = 1.72/0.0718 = 23.96 μCi (886 kBq)

V. BIOLOGICAL HALF-TIMES

A. Exponential Removal

Biological half-lives (T_b), or half-times, as they are also called, assume exponential removals from organs as well as from the whole body. This may not be always correct, but they help us understand the dynamics of radionuclide retention times, internal dosimetry, and risks of radiation injury. With very few exceptions, biological half-times are the same for all isotopes of a given element. See also effective half-lives earlier in this chapter.

Table 9.9 shows the biological half-times of some chemical elements of biological importance. In each case, the critical organ and the whole-body half-time is given. The values shown are average numbers. They can be used to make estimates of retention times, body burdens, and organ burdens.

TABLE 9.9
Biological Half-Times

Element	Whole-Body T_b	Organ	Organ T_b
Calcium	4.5 y	Bone	4.9 y
Chlorine	29 d	Whole body	29 d
Cesium	70 d	Whole body	70 d
Hydrogen	12 d	Whole body	12 d
Iodine	138 d	Thyroid	138 d
Lead	4 y	Kidneys	6 d
Molybdenum	5 d	Kidneys	3 d
Radium	2.2 y	Bone	45 y
Sodium	11 d	Whole body	11 d
Thallium	5 d	Kidneys	1.45 y
Uranium	100 d	Kidneys	15 d

PROBLEMS

Radiopharmaceutical companies include internal dosimetry information in their RP package inserts. For that reason, NMDs, NMPs, and NMTs do not have to do routine internal dose calculations. However, occasionally, they participate in RP research and need to do such calculations. The problems given here can be solved easily using Equation 9.5 and Equation 9.7.

1. Calculate the dose to the thyroid gland from 10 μCi of ^{131}I. Assume 30% gland uptake and an effective half-time of 7 d. The mean absorbed dose (S value) is 2.2×10^{-2} rad/μCi h.
2. Determine the dose to the lungs of a patient who received 5 mCi of ^{99m}Tc-MAA. Assume a 100% uptake and an effective half-time of 5 h. The S value is 5.2×10^{-5}.
3. Assuming that the radiation weighting factor for low-energy negatrons, under 30 keV, is 1.7, convert an absorbed dose of 15 rad to an equivalent dose in sieverts.
4. Calculate the dose to the kidneys from a 2-mCi uptake of ^{99m}Tc-S-colloid in the liver. Assume indefinite retention and an S value liver-to-kidneys of 3.9×10^{-6}.
5. Calculate the dose to the thyroid gland from 100 μCi of ^{123}I iodide given to a patient. Assume 30% uptake and an effective half-time of 12 h. The S value is 4×10^{-3}.
6. Calculate the dose to the kidneys from a 1-mCi uptake of ^{99m}Tc-DMSA. Assume an effective half-time of 2.4 h and an S value of 1.9×10^{4}.
7. Estimate the dose to the fetus from 2 mCi of ^{99m}Tc-MAA in the lungs of a patient. Assume an effective half-time of 5 h and a mean absorbed dose (S value) lungs-to-fetus of 8.4×10^{-8}.

8. Estimate the dose to the whole body from a 25-mCi injection of ^{99m}Tc-MDP given to a patient for skeletal imaging. Tables show that, for a 2-h voiding, the whole-body dose is 6 mrad/mCi.
9. Calculate the total dose to the liver from a 2-mCi uptake of ^{99m}Tc-S-colloid in the liver, a 400-μCi uptake in the spleen, and a 100-μCi uptake in the bone marrow. Assume indefinite retention. The S values are
   4.6×10^{-5} (liver-to-liver)
   9.8×10^{-7} (spleen-to-liver)
   1.6×10^{-6} (bone-marrow-to-liver)
10. Calculate the dose to the bladder wall from an injection of 18 mCi of ^{18}F-FDG given to a patient for PET imaging of malignant disease. The patient voided at 2 h. Table 9.4 shows that, under those conditions, the dose to the bladder wall is 4.4 rads/10 mCi.

REFERENCES

AcutecTM, ^{99m}Tc-Apcitide, package insert by Diatide, Inc., Londonderry, 1998.

Bevalacqua, J.J., *Basic Health Physics — Problems and Solutions*, Wiley–VCH, Weinheim, Germany, 1999.

Bexxar®, ^{131}I-Tositumomab, package insert by GlaxoSmithKline, Research Triangle Park, NC, 2005.

Brix, G. et al., Radiation exposure of patients undergoing whole-body dual-modality ^{18}F-FDG PET/CT examinations, *J. Nucl. Med.*, 46, 608, 2005.

Cardiolite®, ^{99m}Tc-Sestamibi, package insert by Bristol–Myers Squibb, N. Billerica, 2003.

CIS-PyroTM, ^{99m}Tc-Pyrophosphate, package insert by CIS–US, Inc., Bedford, MA, 2005.

CIS-Sulfur ColloidTM, package insert by CIS–US, Inc., Bedford, MA, 2002.

Code of Federal Regulations, Title 10, National Archives Records Administration, Washington, DC, 2005.

DMSA, ^{99m}Tc-Succimer Injection, package insert by Amersham Health, Arlington Heights, VA, 2003.

Drax ImageTM, ^{99m}Tc-Macroaggregated Albumin, package insert by Draximage, Inc., Quebec, 2002.

Early, P.J., *Review of Rules and Regulations Governing the Practice of Nuclear Medicine*, 41st Annual Meeting of the Society of Nuclear Medicine, Orlando, 1994.

Early, P.J. and Sodee, D.B., *Principles and Practice of Nuclear Medicine*, 2d ed., Mosby, St. Louis, 1995.

Fluorodeoxyglucose ^{18}F-FDG Injection, package insert by Eastern Isotopes, Inc., Sterling, VA, 2001.

Gallium citrate Ga-67 Injection, package insert by Bristol-Myers Squibb, N. Billerica, MA, 2003.

Ibritumomab tiuxetan, package insert by IDEC Pharmaceuticals Corporation, San Diego, 2002.

Klingensmith, W.C., Eshima, D., and Goddard, J., *Nuclear Medicine Procedure Manual*, Oxford Medical, Englewood, NJ, 1991.

Kowalsky, R.J. and Falen, S.W., *Radiopharmaceuticals in Nuclear Pharmacy and Nuclear Medicine*, 2d ed., American Pharmacists Association, Washington, DC, 2004.

Landauer, *A Guide to the Personnel Monitoring for Radiation in the Hospital Environment*, Landauer, Glenwood, IL, 2004.

Love, C. and Palestro, C.J., Radionuclide imaging of infection, *J. Nucl. Med. Technol.*, 32, 47, 2004.

Mason, J.S., Elliot, K.M., and Mitro, A.C., *The Nuclear Medicine Handbook for Achieving Compliance with NRC Regulations*, Society of Nuclear Medicine, Reston, VA, 1997.

Metastron®, Strontium-89 Chloride Injection, package insert by Amersham Healthcare, Arlington Heights, VA, 1993.

MDP-Bracco™, ^{99m}Tc-Medronate, package insert by Bracco Diagnostics, Princeton, 2003.

Nagle, C., Editor, New internal radiation dose and modeling software; FDA approves commercial MIRDOSE successor, *J. Nucl. Med.*, 45, 26N, 2004.

Neotec™, ^{99m}Tc-Depreotide, package insert by Diatide, Inc., Londonderry, NH, 1999.

Neuropure, ^{123}I-meta-iodobenzylguanidine, package insert by Nordion International, Inc., Torrance, CA, 2002.

Neutrospec™, ^{99m}Tc-Lanolesomab, package insert by Mallinckrodt, Inc., St. Louis, 2004.

Noz, M.E. and Maguire, G.Q., *Radiation Protection in the Radiologic and Health Sciences*, 2d ed., Lea & Febiger, Philadelphia, 1995.

Octreoscan®, Indium-111-Pentetreotide, package insert by Mallinckrodt, Inc., St. Louis, 2000.

Phosphocol®, Chromic Phosphate Suspension, package insert by Mallinckrodt Inc., St. Louis, 2000.

Saha, G.B., *Physics and Radiobiology of Nuclear Medicine*, Springer–Verlag, New York, 1993.

Saha, G.B., *Basics of PET Imaging*, Springer, New York, 2005.

Shani, G., Radiation Dosimetry — Instrumentation and Methods, 2d ed., CRC Press, Boca Raton, 2000.

Shleien, B., Slaback, Jr., L.A. and Birky, B.K., *Handbook of Health Physics and Radiological Health*, 3d ed., Lippincott Williams & Wilkins, Philadelphia, 1998.

Silverstein, E.B., et al., SNM guidelines for palliative treatment of painful bone metastases in SNM Procedure Guidelines Manual, Society of Nuclear Medicine, Reston, VA, 2003.

SIR-Spheres®, Yttrium-90 Microspheres, package insert by Sirtex Medical, Inc., Lake Forest, IL, 2004.

Spectamine®, ^{123}I-Iofetamine, package insert by Medi-Physics, Inc., Paramus, NJ, 1988.

Stabin, M.G., Proposed addendum to previously published fetal dose estimate tables for ^{18}F-FDG, *J. Nucl. Med.*, 45, 634, 2004.

Technelite®, Mo99/Tc99m Generator, package insert by Bristol–Myers Squibb, N. Billerica, MA, 2003.

Turner, J.A., *Atoms, Radiation, and Radiation Protection*, 2d ed., John Wiley & Sons, New York, 1995.

Ultratag® RBC, package insert by Mallinckrodt, Inc., St. Louis, 2000.

Zanzonico, P.B., Internal radionuclide radiation dosimetry: A review of basic concepts and recent developments, *J. Nucl. Med.*, 41, 297, 2000.

10 Introduction to Radiobiology

I. RATIONALE

Radiobiology is the study of the effects of radiation on biological systems. NM professionals use ionizing radiations in the diagnosis and therapy of many illnesses. Acquiring a basic understanding of radiobiology is essential in the practice of their professions, because they must maximize the benefits of their procedures while minimizing the risks of radiation injury to themselves, to patients, to coworkers, and to the public. They must also understand that their professions involve a small risk of exposure to low levels of radiation over many years of practice. Understanding radiobiology will strengthen the reasons for practicing ALARA. Furthermore, the fundamentals of radiobiology will help clarify the reasons for the protocols used in radionuclide therapy.

This chapter begins with a review of the basic concepts in biology, a description of the sources of radiation, and the methods of observation used in radiobiology. A discussion of the theories of radiation effects on biological systems follows and the reasons why DNA is considered the most sensitive target. The acute radiation syndrome is presented next, followed by a discussion of chronic exposures, the meaning of risks of late effects such as life-span shortening, malignant illness, genetic effects, and the effects of prenatal irradiation.

II. REVIEW OF BASIC CONCEPTS

A. Living Organisms

Living organisms are highly organized chemical systems that comply with the first and second laws of thermodynamics. They are low-entropy systems that (a) must obtain energy from external sources and (b) must have a continuous flow of energy. Upon death, the flow of energy stops, and entropy tends to a maximum.

B. Properties of Living Organisms

Living organisms have four basic properties:

1. Metabolism: This includes all the chemical transformations by which organisms maintain the flow of energy. It is divided into anabolism, the

synthesis of organic compounds, and catabolism, the breakdown of organic compounds.

2. Irritability: This is a short-term biological reaction to changes in the environment. An example is dilatation of the pupils when entering a dark room.
3. Adaptation: This is a long-term response to changes in the environment. Genetic changes come into play. An example is human migrations many thousands of years ago.
4. Reproduction: This is a manifestation of metabolism by which organisms replicate themselves. This results in the survival of the species.

C. Energy Flow

Organisms consist of cells arranged in the form of tissues that make up organ systems. They interact with the environment to obtain and sustain the flow of energy. Some groups are recognized:

1. Green plants: Green plants produce their own food. They use solar energy to synthesize carbohydrates in the process of photosynthesis. They then use those carbohydrates as a source of energy in the process of respiration.

$$\text{Photosynthesis:}\quad 6CO_2 + 12H_2O \longrightarrow \text{Glucose} + 6O_2 + 6H_2O$$

$$\text{Respiration:}\quad \text{Glucose} + 6O_2 \longrightarrow 6CO_2 + 6H_2O + \text{Energy}$$

2. Animals: Animals depend on plants or other animals for food. Plant carbohydrates are used to produce energy by respiration. Proteins and fats are converted into acetate and then used in the same process to produce energy. Animal cells are microscopic. They vary in volume from about 500 to 5000 μm^3 and weigh about the same in picograms. Examples of laboratory animals used in radiobiological research are mice, rats, hamsters, guinea pigs, rabbits, etc. Animals are protected by very strict rules and regulations of animal care prescribed by the National Institutes of Health (NIH) and the National Science Foundation (NSF).
3. Bacteria: Bacteria are plants. They use various pigments to absorb light to produce their own food. They may also resort to symbiosis, commensalism, and parasitism to survive. An example of bacteria used in radiobiological research is *Escherichia coli*.
4. Viruses: Viruses are intermediate between living and nonliving organisms. They can crystallize and remain in a latent state until suitable conditions are found for reproduction. To reproduce, they enter living cells and utilize the host cell metabolic system. Examples are the viruses of the common cold, the virus of poliomyelitis, and the human immunodeficiency virus (HIV).

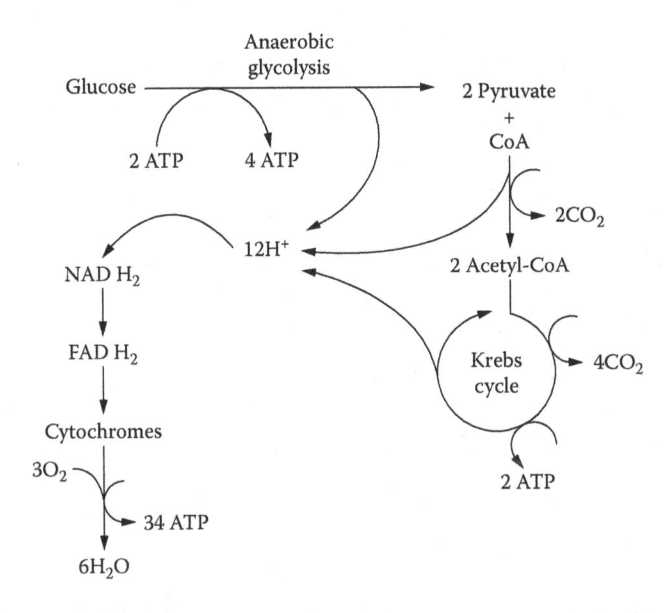

FIGURE 10.1 Cellular respiration and its four reactions: Anaerobic glycolysis (top reaction); aerobic glycolysis: transition reaction (top right); Krebs cycle (bottom right); and electron transport chain (bottom left).

D. Cellular Respiration

Respiration is the process by which glucose is converted into energy. Figure 10.1 is a diagram showing the four basic reactions of cellular respiration. Many enzymes and coenzymes catalyze the reactions: oxidases, dehydrogenases, phosphorylases, adenosine triphosphate (ATP) synthases, oxygenases, decarboxylases, etc. Coenzymes are acetyl coenzyme A (CoA), NAD, FAD, Q coenzyme, cytochromes, etc.

1. Anaeorobic glycolysis: Glucose is converted into two molecules of pyruvate without participation of oxygen, hence the name of anaerobic glycolysis. Two ATPs are used to prime the reaction. In addition to pyruvate, four ATPs are produced. ATP is a high-energy phosphate and contains high-energy chemical bonds. When ATP is converted into adenosine diphosphate (ADP), energy is released. That energy can be used to make many regular chemical bonds in the process of chemical synthesis. For that reason, ATP has been called the *energy currency* of cell metabolism. This first reaction occurs in the cytoplasm.
2. Aerobic glycolysis: In the next three reactions, the breakdown of glucose continues. They occur in the mitochondria. The third reaction ends with the participation of oxygen in the production of metabolic water. For this reason, those reactions are also known as aerobic glycolysis. The three reactions are

a. Transition reaction: In this reaction, pyruvate enters the mitochondria and reacts with CoA, a coenzyme containing pantothenic acid (a vitamin B). In the process, two acetyl-CoAs are produced, and two CO_2 molecules are released.
b. Krebs cycle: The Krebs cycle is also known as the *citric acid cycle,* because one of its reactants is citric acid, and *oxidative decarboxylation* because of its nine oxidation steps and the release of four molecules of CO_2. The cycle produces two more ATPs.
c. Respiratory chain: In this reaction, also known as the *electron transport chain*, 12 hydrogen ions (protons) released in the previous three reactions are transferred along a chain of coenzymes, which are reduced and oxidized in the process while, at the same time, electrons are transferred in the opposite direction. Among those coenzymes, nicotinamide dinucleotide (NAD), flavine adenine dinucleotide (FAD), and a series of cytochromes can be mentioned. Finally, three molecules of oxygen react with the hydrogen to produce six molecules of metabolic water and 34 ATP molecules.

Note: In cases of extreme exertion, such as when running the marathon, the oxygen demand exceeds the oxygen supply. Muscle cells must depend on anaerobic glycolysis for ATPs. The pyruvate produced is quickly converted to lactate, which accumulates in muscles, causing cramps and fatigue.

E. Cell Division

Cell division is the process by which intermitotic tissues maintain their cell populations in dynamic equilibrium. Cells that die are replaced by mitosis. In this process, two types of cells must be recognized:

1. Somatic cells: Somatic cells constitute most body tissues. Cell renewal depends on mitosis. In humans, each parent cell produces two daughter cells, each containing 23 pairs of chromosomes. After approximately 50 cell divisions, some cells die by apoptosis (DNA-programmed death) and equilibrium is maintained.
2. Germinal cells: These are the spermatogonia and oogonia that undergo a process of cell division and maturation known as meiosis. In this process, cells reduce their chromosomes to 23 (one member of each pair) and reshuffle their genes by crossing over. Each spermatogonium produces four viable sperm cells. Each oogonia produces one viable oocyte and three nonviable cells.

F. Mitosis

For most intermitotic tissues, mitosis lasts about 1 h and consists of four phases. Under the microscope, each phase can be recognized by

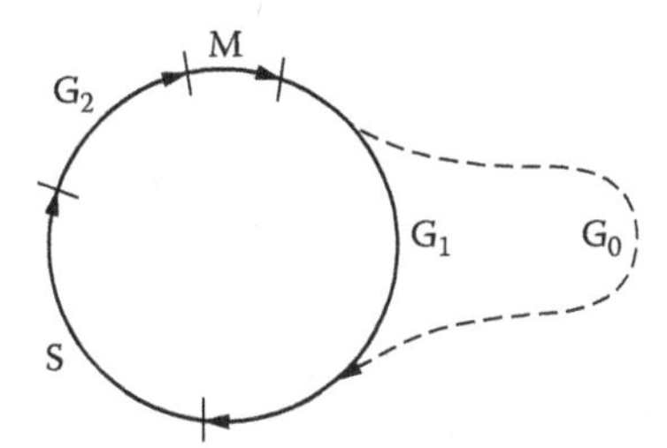

FIGURE 10.2 The cell cycle of an intermitotic tissue and its four stages: mitosis (M), gap 1 (G_1), DNA synthesis (S), and gap 2 (G_2). The latent stage (G_0) of reverting postmitotic tissues is also shown.

1. *Prophase*: Filamentous DNA organizes into chromosomes, the nuclear membrane dissolves, and the spindle forms.
2. *Metaphase*: Guided by the spindle, the chromosomes are arranged in the equatorial plane of the cell. They thicken and divide longitudinally into two chromatids.
3. *Anaphase*: Chromatids separate and are guided by the spindle toward the polar regions of the cell.
4. *Telophase*: The cell divides into two daughter cells, the nucleus is reconstructed, and the new chromosomes resolve into filamentous DNA.

Cells that are not dividing are said to be in "interphase."

G. The Cell Cycle

The life cycle of cells has been studied using radioisotopes (radiotracers), flow cytometry, and time-lapse movies. Figure 10.2 shows a typical cell cycle with its four stages:

1. Mitosis (M): In this stage, cells divide as described above.
2. Gap 1 (G_1): Cells prepare for DNA replication.
3. DNA synthesis (S): DNA doubles by replication.
4. Gap 2 (G_2): Cells prepare for mitosis.

For most tissues, the duration of the cycle varies from 18 to 48 h depending on the duration of G_1, the most variable stage. In some differentiated tissues (reverting postmitotic), cells may enter a latent state called G_0. For example, in the adult liver, most hepatocytes perform all normal functions except mitosis. In emergencies such as trauma, hepatocytes return to a very active mitosis to regenerate the lost tissue.

H. Defense Mechanisms

In humans and laboratory animals, the organism is protected by a series of barriers against physical, chemical, and biological agents capable of causing illness. Those barriers are

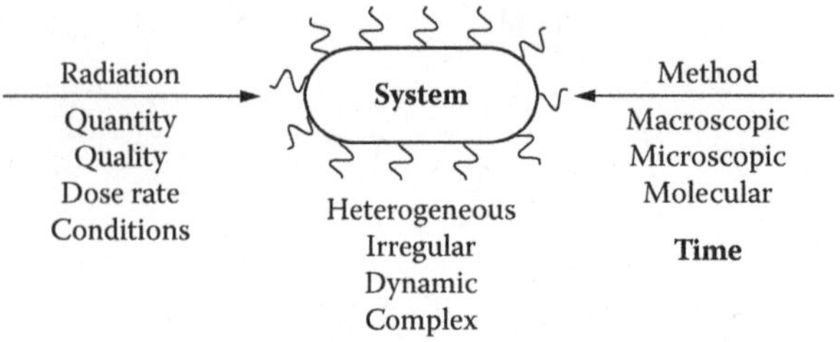

Radiation
Quantity
Quality
Dose rate
Conditions

System
Heterogeneous
Irregular
Dynamic
Complex

Method
Macroscopic
Microscopic
Molecular
Time

FIGURE 10.3 The study of radiobiology and its three components: the radiation source (left), the biological system (center), and the method of observation (right).

1. Primary barriers: Represented by the skin and mucosal membranes of the GI, respiratory, and urogenital systems.
2. Secondary barriers: These are the network of lymphatic vessels and the regional lymphatic glands. They represent the "third circulation," the lymph.
3. Tertiary barriers: Represented by all fixed and migrant cells of the reticuloendothelial system (RES). Among them are the Kupffer cells of the liver, the reticular cells of the spleen, the bone marrow, and the lymphatic glands, the macrophages and the mast cells of connective tissues, the leukocytes of the blood, and the glial cells of the nervous tissues.

III. THE STUDY OF RADIOBIOLOGY

A. The General Scheme

Figure 10.3 shows diagrammatically the approach used in radiobiological research. On one side is the source of radiation used: alpha, beta, gamma, x-rays, neutrons, protons, deuterons, pi-mesons, etc. In the center is the biological system: a complex organism, virus, bacteria, plant, or animal. On the other side is the method of observation: macroscopic, microscopic, molecular, and subatomic. The radiation effects observed and how soon they are observed depend largely on the method of observation used.

B. Sources of Radiation

The human population is exposed constantly to natural and artificial sources of radiation. In the United States, the breakdown of average annual radiation doses is shown in Table 10.1.

1. Natural sources: By far, radon is the largest natural source, accounting for 55% of the total dose to the public. Terrestrial radiation comes from trace amounts of ^{238}U, ^{232}Th, their products of decay, and other radionuclides present in the ground and construction materials. Secondary cosmic radiation consists of showers of particles produced by collisions of primary cosmic radiation coming from the sun and the stars with the upper

TABLE 10.1
Sources of Radiation

	Percentage	(mrem/y)	(mSv/y)
	Natural (82%)		
Radon	55	198	1.98
Terrestrial	8	29	0.29
Cosmic	8	29	0.29
Internal	11	39	0.39
	Artificial (18%)		
X-rays	11	39	0.39
Nuclear medicine	4	14	0.14
Consumer products	3	11	0.11
Other	<1	3	0.03
Total	**100**	**362**	**3.62**

layers of the atmosphere. Internal radiation is mostly from ^{40}K and some ^{14}C and ^{3}H present in nature and all living organisms.

2. Artificial sources: Artificial radiations come from medical, nuclear, and other industries and their products. Artificial radiations represent only 18% of the total radiation dose; 82% comes from natural sources.
3. Levels of radiation: Radiobiologists use radiation sources at two very distinct levels:
   a. Low level, as radiotracers, in which minute amounts of radioactive nuclides are used to "trace" the physiopathology of biological systems without altering them. Examples are diagnostic NM procedures.
   b. High level, as sources of energy, in which large amounts of radiation are used to change the irradiated system purposely. Examples are radiation therapy and radionuclide therapy of malignant illnesses.

C. The Biological System

1. Systems studied: Depending on the scientific background of the radiobiologist, the systems used may be viruses, bacteria, plants, insects, or laboratory animals. Living tissues might be studied *in vivo* (in the whole animal), or *in vitro* (in petri dishes or bottles). Animals can be mice, hamsters, rats, rabbits, or farm animals. Animals under experimentation are protected by very strict standards of animal care.
2. Experimental design: The experimental design always includes two groups of subjects chosen at random: the experimental group subjected to irradiation and the control group subjected to exactly the same conditions of the other group except irradiation. In this fashion, the differences between the two groups are attributed to radiation. Careful design and observations of the control group are a way to make progress in understanding physiology.

3. Conditions: The effects observed after irradiation also depend on the conditions before, during, and after irradiation. For example, irradiation at room temperature vs. irradiation in the frozen state, irradiation in the aerated state vs. irradiation under hypoxia, presence vs. absence of a chemotherapeutic drug, etc.
4. The method of observation: Besides the quality and quantity of radiation, the degree of sophistication in the method of observation is a deciding factor in what will be observed and how soon it will be observed.

IV. TYPES OF EXPOSURE

For didactic purposes, two types of exposure are considered: acute and chronic. They are described briefly next.

A. Acute Exposure

A high dose of radiation is delivered within a short time, for example, several hundreds or even thousands of rems (a few Gy to many Gy) delivered over a few seconds or minutes. This type of exposure results in deterministic effects, which means that the severity of the effect increases with the dose given to the system under study. In radiation therapy and radionuclide therapy, acute irradiations are used to destroy malignant tissues, but those exposures are restricted to the malignant tissues with minimal exposure of the rest of the body.

Figure 10.4(b) shows a typical curve for deterministic effects: threshold nonlinear with saturation at higher doses. For example, the acute radiation syndrome (ARS), observed accidentally in humans and experimentally in laboratory animals, is described later in this chapter.

To prevent accidental acute exposures, radiation workers must apply and enforce safety rules at all times in all nuclear reactor facilities, accelerator facilities, food-irradiation plants, industrial radiography operations, and in hospitals, clinics (radiology and nuclear medicine), and dental offices (dental radiology).

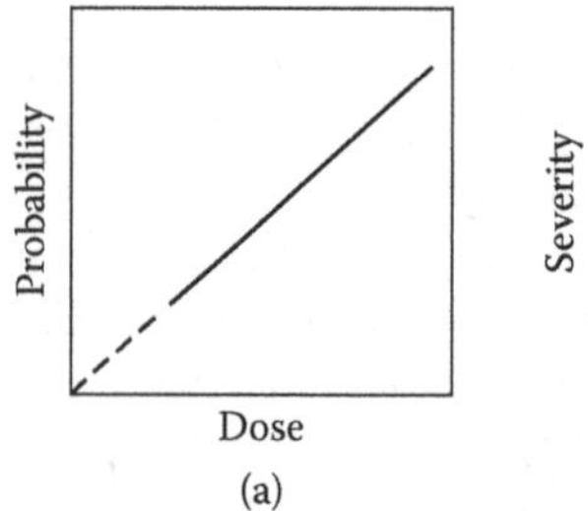

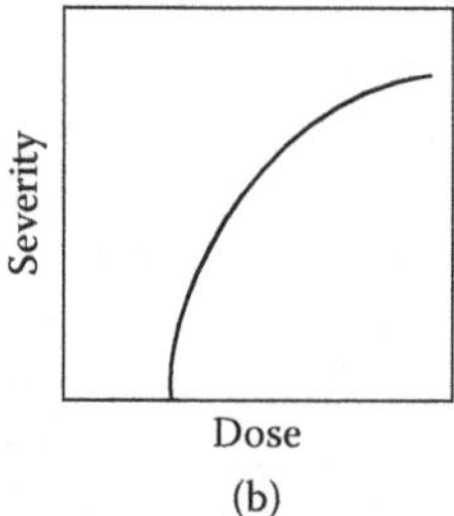

FIGURE 10.4 Types of late effects: (a) stochastic, in which the probability of observing the effect increases with dose, (b) deterministic, in which the severity of the effect increases with dose.

B. Chronic Exposure

A low dose of radiation is delivered over a long time. A few rems or millirems (a few μSv to a few mSv) are delivered over many days or weeks or even years. Chronic exposures result in stochastic effects, which means that the probability of observing the effect increases with the dose given. A graph of probability vs. dose may result in the straight line shown in Figure 10.4(a).

Examples of chronic exposures are background radiation and occupational exposure of radiation workers. To minimize low-level exposures of radiation workers, ALARA must be practiced at all times.

C. Experimental Levels of Exposure

In general, in experimental mammalian radiobiology, three dose ranges are recognized:

1. Low level: Less than 100 rem (1 Sv); expected for whole-body irradiation with x- or gamma rays: mild illness, 100% survival.
2. Moderate level: 100 to 500 rem (1 to 5 Sv); expected for whole-body irradiation with x- or gamma rays: mild to severe illness; recovery likely. The lethal dose 50% within 30 d, $LD_{50/30}$, for most laboratory animals varies between 300 to 500 rem (3 to 5 Sv).
3. High level: More than 500 rem (more than 5 Sv); expected: severe illness. Without medical treatment, recovery is unlikely.

V. THEORIES OF RADIATION INJURY

A. Introduction

Two theories have prevailed over the years to explain the effects of irradiation in biological systems. Figure 10.5 is a diagram that presents the theories.

1. Direct theory: The direct action theory or target theory considers that the energy of radiation causes changes in specific and vital cell targets. Targets may be DNA, RNA, enzymes, hormones, organelles (mitochondria, ribosomes, and lysosomes), and internal or external membranes.
2. Indirect theory: The indirect action theory considers that the radiation energy interacts with the most abundant substance in cells: water, a polar solvent, producing many molecular fragments, radicals, and ions that react with each other and with everything else in cells. Some of the recombination products, such as free radicals (FRs) and hydrogen peroxide (H_2O_2), are powerful oxidants and toxic to specific targets within cells. All this comprehends the physical, prechemical, and chemical stages of the theory and lasts less than 1 μs.
3. The biological stage: The biological stage is common to both theories and may last from milliseconds to years, and depends largely on the sensitivity of the system and the conditions during irradiation. Most of the observed

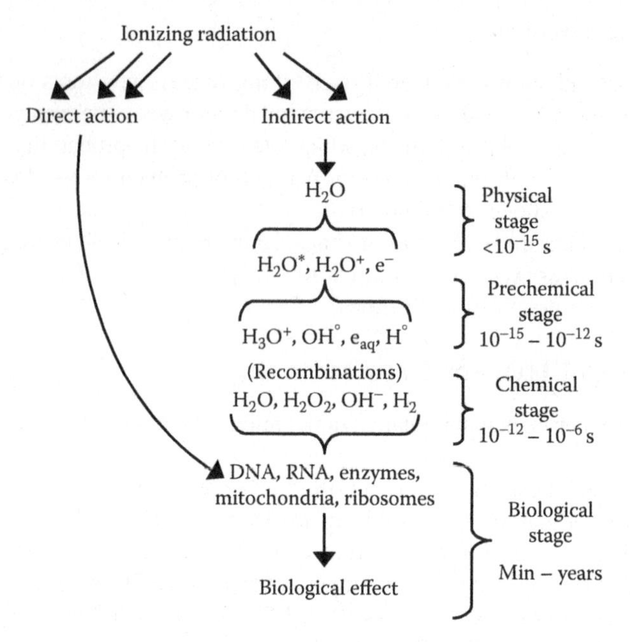

FIGURE 10.5 Theories of direct and indirect actions. In the direct action theory, the energy of the radiation acts directly on specific cell targets. In the indirect action theory, the breakdown of water and the recombination of its products cause changes in cell targets.

effects are a combination of direct and indirect actions. In most cases, cell inactivation means reproductive death or the inability to divide.

B. Target Theory

The target theory is demonstrated with biophysical, biochemical, and viral systems in the dry state. The required evidence is as follows:

1. The effect is an exponential function of dose.
2. The effect is independent of dose rate.
3. The effect is proportional to ion density.

Figure 10.6 is an example of a target theory effect. The surviving fraction is plotted against radiation dose. The curve is exponential. Graph (a) is a plot on linear graph paper. Graph (b) is the same on semilogarithmic graph paper. The equation for the curve is

$$S = e^{-D/D_0} \tag{10.1}$$

where S = surviving fraction, D = dose given, and D_0 = dose required to inactivate all targets; also known as the 37% dose.

Owing to the exponential nature of the curve, when D = D_0, only 63% of the targets are inactivated and 37% survive. This is because $e^{-1} = 0.37$.

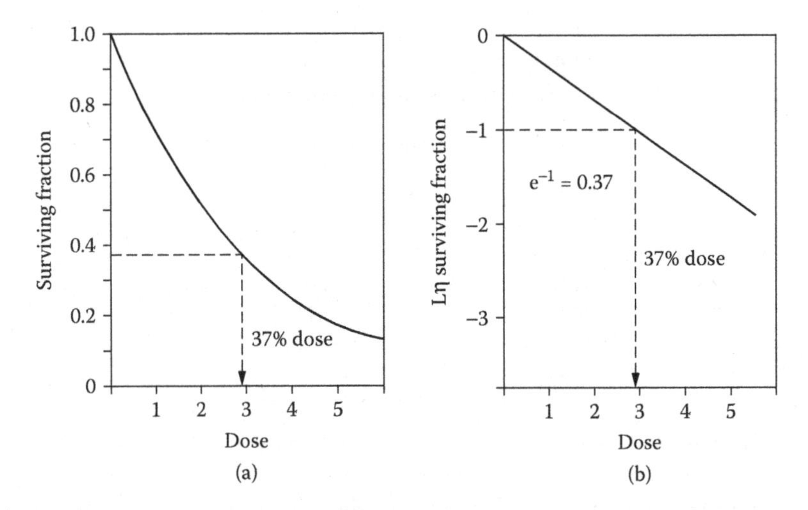

FIGURE 10.6 Direct (target) theory. The effect is an exponential function of dose ((a), linear graph; (b), semilogarithmic graph). On both, the 37% dose is indicated.

C. Indirect Theory

In the prechemical stage, free radicals OH^O (hydroxyl), H^O (atomic hydrogen), and hydrated electrons (e_{aq}) are produced. Free radicals (FRs) are responsible for the inactivation of important molecules in cells. Some properties of FRs are

1. They have an unpaired electron. That makes them very reactive. They stick to any molecule, rendering it inactive.
2. They are neutral. Figure 10.7 shows the difference between a hydroxyl FR (neutral) and a hydroxyl ion (negatively charged). Another example is atomic hydrogen, which is neutral and has an unpaired electron (H^O).

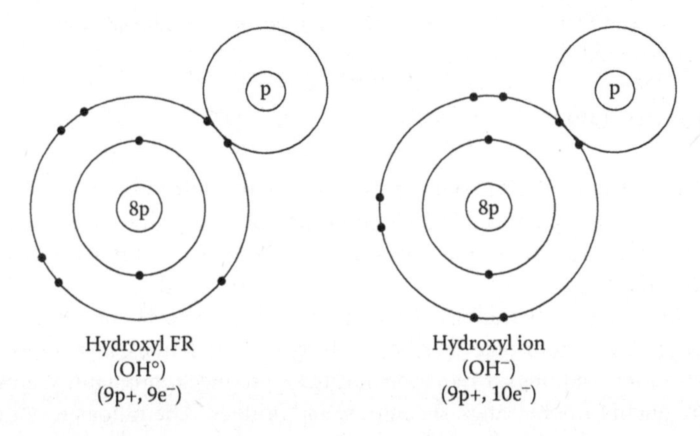

FIGURE 10.7 The difference between the hydroxyl free radical (neutral) and the hydroxyl ion (negatively charged) is shown.

TABLE 10.2
Composition of a Human Cell

Substance	Number of Molecules/Cell
DNA	46
RNA	202
Proteins	32,200
Lipids	322,000
Other, organic	184,000
Inorganic	3,220,000
Water	552,000,000

3. Because they are very reactive, they travel only about 30 Å (3×10^{-9} m) or so before interacting with some molecule.
4. For the same reason, they have very short lives of less than 1 μs.
5. They can be detected by electron spin resonance (ESR).

Approximately two thirds of body weight is water. This is true for all vertebrates, even fish. Approximately 70 to 90% of cells is water. Table 10.2 gives the approximate composition of an average human cell.

The data in Table 10.2 shows that water is the most abundant substance and, consequently, the most probable target. Proteins and lipids can be disrupted to some extent, and the cell will recover. On the other hand, DNA and RNA disruptions can be catastrophic to cell survival.

VI. DNA: THE MOST SENSITIVE TARGET

Because 1 Sv (100 rem) of ionizing radiation can produce 6.1×10^{13} ionizations/g of tissue, and because each cell contains 4×10^{-12} g of DNA, 1 Sv can produce 244 ionizations in the DNA of each cell, or 5.3 ionizations per chromosome. No wonder DNA is considered the most sensitive target.

A. Lesions in DNA

1. The G value: The G value is the number of molecules changed by 100 eV of energy spent. Table 10.3 gives G values for various lesions in DNA. Other lesions are strand cross-linking, protein cross-linking, and base dimerization.
2. Chromosome aberrations: Irradiation during stage G_1 of the cell cycle produces chromosome aberrations: fragments, deletions, inversions, translocations, and rings. Irradiation during G_2 produces chromatid aberrations: fragments, double rings, dicentrics, and bridges. Aberrations result in cell inactivation and reproductive death.

TABLE 10.3
Molecular Lesions in DNA

Molecular Change	G Value[a]
Release of phosphate	0.09
Double-strand break	0.12
Release of ammonia	0.47
Sugar-phosphate rupture	2.0
Single-strand break	2–10
H-bond breakage	50–60

[a] Number of Molecules changed/100 eV.

B. Role of DNA

1. Chromosomes: A chromosome is a very involved molecule of DNA. The molecular weight of a chromosome in animal cells varies between 1 and 10 billion daltons (Da). Human chromosomes average about 3 billion Da. Figure 10.8 is a diagram of a portion of a chromosome. Proteins called histones bind and coat the DNA molecule.
2. Structure: Double-stranded DNA is made of two polynucleotide chains. Each nucleotide contains deoxyribose, phosphate, and a base (purine or pyrimidine). The two chains spiral around each other. The bases in one chain bind bases in the other chain by hydrogen bonds: adenine (A) always binds thymine (T), and cytosine (C) always binds guanine (G). The sequences of base pairs spell gene codes for many protein syntheses and other functions.
3. Genes: In humans, the genome consists of 20,000 to 25,000 genes. Genes contain between 3,000 and 2.4 million base pairs. Each somatic cell has 46

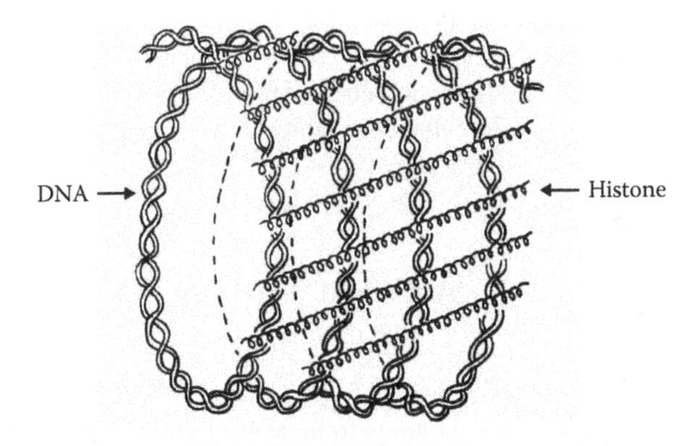

FIGURE 10.8 Artist's conception of a chromosome: a very involved molecule of DNA bound and coated by proteins called histones.

chromosomes. Messenger RNA, ribosomal RNA, and transfer RNA play a role in the synthesis of proteins by various cells in tissues. Proteins function as enzymes, hormones, growth factors, growth inhibitors, etc. in the development, function, adaptation, repair, and metabolism of cells and organisms.

4. Repair of DNA: DNA is constantly exposed to physically, chemically, and biologically harmful agents in the external as well as in the internal environment. Repair of that damage is essential to cell survival. One mechanism of repair involves molecular lesions such as thymine dimers, which can be excised and repaired by enzyme systems containing excinucleases and polymerases. In those cases, the good strand serves as a template for the opposite strand during repair. Failure or insufficiency of the repair mechanisms results in cell death or reproductive cell inactivation.

VII. QUANTITATIVE RADIOBIOLOGY

A. Survival Curves

Puck and Marcus introduced the first survival curves for irradiated human cells in 1952. Survival curves allowed radiobiologists the opportunity to measure cell sensitivities and to compare experiments performed at different locations.

B. Microscopic Autoradiography

At just about the same time, the use of photographic emulsions permitted radiobiologists to "trace" molecules inside cells and to measure molecular renewal rates and turnover. The use of tritiated thymidine permitted the study of the cell cycle and the measurement of the rate of DNA synthesis.

C. Other Methods

Today, radiobiologists have new technologies such as flow cytometry, gel chromatography, gel electrophoresis, and their associated computerized systems. With them, chromosomes can be measured and identified; genes can be identified; and DNA and genes can be produced in significant quantities by the polymerase chain reaction (PCR) using automatic electronic machines and robotics. Proteins can be designed and synthesized in appreciable quantities. Both DNA and proteins can be analyzed overnight using special microanalytical techniques.

VIII. SURVIVAL CURVES

A. Definition

Survival curves are quantitative methods to measure radiobiological effects. They consist of a graph of the surviving fraction on a logarithmic scale vs. the dose given on a linear scale. For most mammalian cells *in vitro*, high-LET radiations yield a straight line. For low-LET radiations, the curve shows a shoulder at low

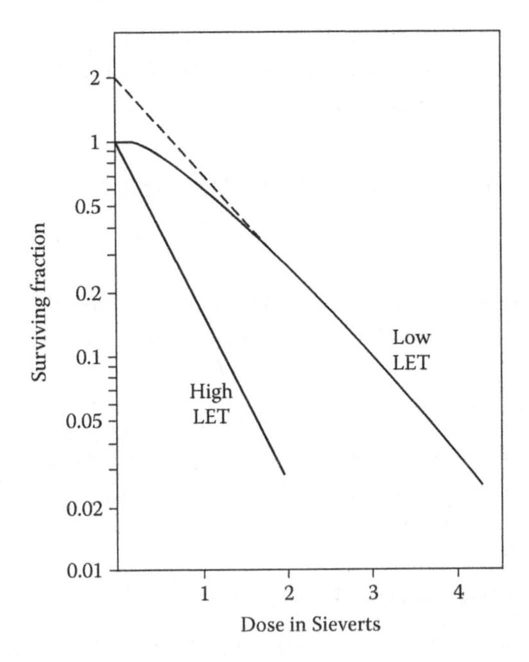

FIGURE 10.9 Survival curves for mammalian cells in culture. Two curves are shown, one resulting from irradiation with a high-LET radiation and another with low-LET radiation. Also shown is the extrapolated number of the second curve.

doses and becomes straight at high doses. The slope of the straight portion of the curve is an expression of the sensitivity of the system under the conditions of the experiment. Figure 10.9 shows the curves for low- and high-LET radiations on mammalian cells *in vitro*.

B. Equations

The equation for the high-LET curve is the same as Equation 10.1 shown above. The equation for low-LET radiations is as follows:

$$S = 1 - (1 - e^{-D/D_0})^n \tag{10.2}$$

where S = surviving fraction, e = base of natural logarithms (2.71828...), D = dose given, D_0 = 37% dose, and n = extrapolation number.

C. The Shoulder

Two interpretations have been proposed for the shoulder of the low-LET curves:

1. For inactivation, cells may require that two or more sensitive targets be hit by radiation. The extrapolation number (n) is the number of targets. In Figure 10.9, the extrapolation number for the low-LET curve is 2.

2. At low doses, the cellular mechanisms of repair come into play. That results in greater survival. At high doses, repair is less likely, and the curve becomes a straight line.

IX. TISSUE SENSITIVITIES

A. Cells

All individual cells in culture have the same inherent sensitivity: The LD_{50} (lethal dose 50%) is about 100 rem or 1 Sv. The D_0 is about 130 rem or 1.3 Sv.

B. Cell Populations

Cell populations, on the other hand, have variable sensitivities depending largely on their cell renewal rates. Fast-renewing cells are much more sensitive (steeper survival curves) than slow-renewing cells.

C. The Law of Bergonie and Tribondeau

The law of Bergonie and Tribondeau states that the sensitivity of a tissue is directly proportional to its reproductive activity and inversely proportional to its degree of differentiation. This is true for most tissues with very few exceptions. Tissues with high renewal rates, such as the bone marrow, the intestinal mucosa, the basal layer of the epidermis, the lymphatic tissues, and the stem cells of the germinal tissues are extremely sensitive to radiation. Tissues with very low cell renewal rate such as the neurons, adult hepatocytes, skeletal muscle fibers, cardiac muscle fibers, the adrenal cortex cells, etc. are much less sensitive to radiation. The degree of differentiation refers to the degree of anatomical and physiological sophistication. A very notable exception to the law is the lymphocyte population, which is highly differentiated and yet extremely sensitive.

X. TYPES OF DAMAGE

Three types of damage are recognized: lethal damage, which is irreversible, sublethal damage (SLD), which is repairable within 2 h after irradiation, and potentially lethal damage (PLD), which depends on the conditions after irradiation.

A. Sublethal Damage (SLD)

The shoulder of the low-LET survival curves is said to represent the repair of sublethal damage that occurs at low doses. This repair has been demonstrated using the "split-dose" technique. A gradient of radiation doses is delivered in two halves. Controls receive the same doses in a single exposure. If the interval is less than 2 h, survival is higher than in the control group, meaning that repair has occurred.

B. Potentially Lethal Damage (PLD)

PLD has been demonstrated by comparing survival curves of irradiated cells under normal conditions and the same for cells subjected to some physical or chemical stress after irradiation. Tissues under stress performed better: higher survival. Examples of the stresses applied were

1. Starvation: The nutrient medium was replaced with saline solution after irradiation.
2. Overcrowding: Replanting of cultures was delayed after irradiation.
3. Growth inhibitors: Adding cyclohexamide, a protein synthesis inhibitor, to the cultures after irradiation.

XI. RADIATION INJURY MODIFIERS

A. Physical Modifiers

The most important physical modifiers are

1. Linear energy transfer (LET): A property of the type of radiation, expressed in keV/μm of tissue.
2. Dose rate: The rate at which radiation is delivered to tissues, usually expressed in rem/min or Sv/min. In general, high-LET radiations are more effective than low-LET radiations at inactivating cells *in vitro*. Similarly, high dose rates are more efficient at inactivating cells *in vitro* than low dose rates. This is because low rates allow repair of radiation injury. In x- or gamma-beam therapy of malignant disease, a typical dose rate is 1 Sv/min (100 rem/min).

B. Chemical Modifiers

A most outstanding chemical sensitizer of tissues to radiation is oxygen. Very low levels of oxygen do sensitize tissues. Many drugs used in chemotherapy are either sensitizers of malignant tissues or protectors of normal tissues.

1. The oxygen effect: Oxygen enhances radiation effects. The enhancement is measured by the oxygen enhancement ratio (OER):

$$OER = \frac{\text{Survival under Hypoxia}}{\text{Survival under Aereated Conditions}}$$

For low-LET radiations, the OER varies between 2.5 and 3.0, which means that in the presence of oxygen, x- or gamma rays are 250 to 300% more effective at inactivating tissues than the same under hypoxia. Irradiations with high-LET radiations result in an OER equal to one, which means no enhancement. An explanation for the oxygen effect is that oxygen fixes free radicals by reacting with them. The toxic oxidants produced, such as hydrogen peroxide (a bleacher), are extremely effective at inactivating cells *in vitro*. Antioxidants such as vitamin C and vitamin E reduce the amount of FRs produced and consequently reduce also the amount of peroxide.

2. Other chemical modifiers: Some drugs alter radiation effects. Protectors reduce effects in normal tissues. Sensitizers enhance effects in abnormal tissues. Five groups are recognized:
   a. *True protectors*: Reducing agents, such as cysteine, cysteamine, and cystamine, which react with FRs. For that reason, they are called *FR scavengers*.
   b. *Pseudoprotectors*: These reduce radiation effects by altering metabolism. Examples are epinephrine, histamine, and carbon monoxide.
   c. *True sensitizers*: These substances become incorporated into the DNA molecule of tumoral cells, rendering them more susceptible to radiation. Examples are 5-Cl-deoxyuridine and 5-Br-deoxycytidine.
   d. *Pseudosensitizers*: These compounds sensitize by altering metabolism. Examples are the antitumor antibiotics actinomycin, bleomycin, adriamycin, and methotrexate.
   e. *Sensitizers of hypoxic cells*: Hypoxic cells in solid, nonvascularized tumors are responsible for tumor recurrence after therapy. Examples of such tumors are the squamous cell carcinoma of the skin and the bronchogenic carcinoma of the lungs. Sensitizers of hypoxic cells, such as nitroimidazoles, are used along with radiation in a more effective therapy of those tumors.

C. Biological Modifiers

The relative biological effectiveness (RBE) is the ratio of the effectiveness of various types of radiations (neutrons, protons, pi-mesons, etc.) with that of x- or gamma rays at destroying malignant tissues. The formula is

$$\text{RBE} = \frac{\text{Dose of X- or Gamma Rays} \rightarrow \text{Effect}}{\text{Dose of Other Radiation} \rightarrow \text{Same Effect}}$$

RBEs depend on the end point of the effect. For example, for human cancer cells (HeLa cells) *in vitro*, the RBE at 80% survival is shown in Table 10.4. HeLa is an abbreviation of Helen Larks, the name of the woman from whom the original uterine cancer cells were taken and cultured for experimental research.

D. The Overkill Effect

RBEs increase with LET up to 100 keV/μm. Beyond that, RBEs decrease. That is, LETs higher than 100 keV/μm represent wasted dose, and may cause unnecessary harm to normal tissues surrounding the tumor.

TABLE 10.4
RBEs for HeLa Cells at 80% Survival

Radiation	LET (keV/μm)	RBE
X- or γ-rays	1	1.0
Fast neutrons	12	2.6
Alpha rays	100	7.7

E. Dose Fractionation

Delivering the total radiation dose in fractions has proven to be a most effective therapy. The reasons are described as the "four Rs" of radiotherapy.

1. *Redistribution*: The first dose fraction destroys cells in mitosis. Cells then continue their cycle. A second fraction destroys cells entering mitosis. The process is repeated until the complete dose has been delivered. Success depends on proper timing of the fractions.
2. *Reoxygenation*: The first dose fraction destroys many well-oxygenated cells. In the interim, hypoxic cells reoxygenate. A second fraction destroys those. Several fractions, properly timed, result in effective therapy.
3. *Regeneration*: Undifferentiated malignant tissues have a fast regeneration rate. Dose fractionation timed to their specific cell renewal rate can result in effective therapy.
4. *Repair*: Some malignant tumors can be treated more effectively if higher doses are delivered at each fraction. They appear to be less capable of repair under those conditions.

XII. ACUTE RADIATION SYNDROME (ARS)

A. Whole-Body Exposure

1. An acute whole-body exposure to penetrating radiation results in the acute radiation syndrome (ARS). The ARS has been studied in animals with very similar results to those observed in humans after accidental exposure to moderate and high doses of radiation.
2. Various agencies have studied acute exposures in humans and reported a range of $LD_{50/30}$ (lethal dose 50% within 30 d) between 250 and 400 rem (2.5 to 4.0 Sv). An average of seven reports yielded 308 ± 56 rem (3.08 ± 0.56 Sv).
3. The severity of the signs and symptoms of the ARS depend on the magnitude of the dose (deterministic effect with a threshold of about 20 rem or 0.20 Sv). For young adults, the expected clinical conditions are listed in Table 10.5.

TABLE 10.5
Illness from Whole-Body Acute Exposure

Dose (mrem)	(Sv)	Expected Clinical Conditions
Less than 20	(<0.2)	No symptoms (late effects)
20	(0.2)	Threshold for illness
20–100	(0.2–1.0)	ARS, mild illness
100	(1.0)	Threshold for deaths
100–1000	(1.0–10)	ARS, bone marrow syndrome
1000–10,000	(10–100)	ARS, GI syndrome
More than 10,000	(>100)	ARS, CNS syndrome

B. The Bone Marrow Syndrome

Laboratory rats exposed acutely to 750 rem (7.5 Sv) of whole-body irradiation with ^{60}Co gamma rays showed the following signs and symptoms two weeks after irradiation: loss of weight, pallor, anorexia, asthenia, and petechial hemorrhages on the skin. The packed cell volume (PCV) had dropped to 64% of controls, the RBC count was 4.7 million/µl (75% of controls). The leukocyte count was 900/µl (15% of controls). Internally, the animals showed petechial hemorrhages in the subcutaneous tissues and under the peritoneum of abdominal organs. The whole carcass was anemic, and the mesenteric lymphatic glands were hemorrhagic. The spleen weight was only 40% of that of control animals.

Other changes reported in the literature indicate a drop in the lymphocyte count to 3% of controls in 24 h, leukocyte count to 6% of controls in 3 d, platelet count to 23% of controls in 12 d, and RBC count to 56% of controls by the 18th day. The degree of depression of the various blood cell lines appears to be related to their respective cell renewal rates and cell life spans in the circulation. For example, in humans, most lymphocytes live only 1 d in the circulation. If their stem cells in the bone marrow are destroyed by irradiation, there are no replacements by the end of their life spans. Thus, the lymphocytes essentially disappear overnight from the peripheral circulation. The same seems to occur with the granulocytes, whose life spans are about 7 d, the platelets, with life spans of 7 to 10 d, and the erythrocytes, with an approximate 100-d life span. Consequences of the various cell line losses are as follows: loss of leukocytes, increased susceptibility to infections; loss of lymphocytes, immunosuppression; loss of platelets, generalized hemorrhages; and loss of erythrocytes, or anemia. Surviving animals recover gradually over the following three months.

C. GI Syndrome

Reports describe the GI syndrome as follows: with doses around and above 1000 rem (10 Sv), the animals cease eating and drinking water. They lose condition rapidly and feel very ill. The mucosal lining of the GI tract falls apart (denudation), exposing the submucosa. There is massive rupture of capillaries, arterioles, and venules, leading to generalized hemorrhages and hypotension. The severe inflammation and hemorrhages in the GI tract result in distention, pain, and diarrhea. Within 4 d, the life span of the mucosal cells, there is septicemia, circulatory shock, coma, and death. Injury to the bone marrow is severe, but it is secondary to the GI clinical observations.

D. CNS Syndrome

The neurons constitute the parenchyma of the central nervous system (CNS). They are highly differentiated and, in the adult, do not divide at all. According to the law of Bergonie and Tribondeau, they should have a very low sensitivity to radiation. Indeed, they are the least sensitive cells of the body. On the other hand, the supporting tissues in the CNS, the stroma, consisting of blood vessels, lymphatics, glial cells, and connective tissues, have a medium sensitivity and, therefore, are more sensitive than the neurons. A moderate-to-high dose of radiation to the brain is very harmful to its capillary circulation and, consequently, to the neurons.

Experiments with laboratory animals have shown that a dose of 50 Sv delivered to the head only results in massive edema, incoordination, ataxia, stupor, cardiovascular shock, and death. With doses of 1 to 2 Sv to the head, animals recover, and one year later, microscopic examinations show arteriolosclerosis, multiple microaneurysms, and microstrokes.

With doses of 10 to 50 Sv, given to the whole body, the same symptoms mentioned above are observed, but death occurs much sooner, within 24 to 48 h.

E. Radiation Dispersion Device (RDD)

1. Defining the emergency: A radiation dispersion device, also called a “dirty bomb,” is an explosive contraption that could be used by terrorists to spread radioactivity over a populated area. People in that area would be contaminated externally and internally. Radiation emergency agencies need to be prepared to qualify and quantify the radionuclides involved and their chemical nature, to determine the degree of contamination of each person in that area, to register each person, and to send those who need medical treatment to the appropriate location.
2. Personnel: Health physicists, radiation physicists, radiochemists, nuclear physicians, medical physicists, NMTs, radiology technologists, radiation therapy technologists, emergency medical technologists, and nurses are best suited to provide assistance in such an emergency.
3. External contamination: The quickest and most effective way to remove external contamination would be showering with soap and water. Depending on the type of contamination, clothing may have to be discarded as radioactive waste.
4. Internal contamination: Persons who exceed one ALI (annual limit of intake) would be eligible for treatment for internal contamination. Some examples of medical treatment follow:

a. Dilution with stable compounds: Stable iodide or perchlorate given immediately to block the thyroid gland in cases of ^{131}I or ^{125}I contamination.
b. Chelation: Chelating agents such as EDTA or DTPA combine with heavy metals, rendering them soluble in water and thus facilitating their urinary excretion. This treatment would be recommended in cases of uranium or plutonium contamination.
c. Diuretics and water: That treatment would accelerate the urinary excretion of some soluble radionuclides such as ^{137}Cs and ^{3}H (tritium).
d. Prussian blue: Blue dye prescribed in cases of ^{137}Cs contamination.
e. Oral calcium: Prescribed to assist in the removal of ^{222}Ra, ^{226}Ra, and ^{90}Sr.
f. Phosphate: To assist in the removal of ^{32}P.

XIII. LATE EFFECTS OF RADIATION

Individuals exposed to low levels of radiation over a long period of time, as well as individuals who receive an acute sublethal dose of radiation and recover, will eventually show late effects also referred to as delayed effects of radiation. Radiation effects are not characterized by pathognomonic (unique, distinctive) lesions. Lesions found in exposed individuals are the same found in other pathological conditions.

A. Types of Late Effects

1. Stochastic effects: Stochastic effects are statistical in nature. The probability of observing the effects are proportional to the dose of radiation received. For this reason, and because their numbers are usually very low, they can only be studied by statistical methods. Examples are radiation-induced cancers, leukemias, and genetic effects.
2. Deterministic effects: These effects follow a threshold, nonlinear relationship to dose. Examples are erythema, cataracts, and temporary infertility.

Genetic conditions are important regarding the susceptibility to some late effects. Environmental conditions before, during, and after exposure also play a role on the incidence and timing of the late effects observed. Extreme care in statistical sampling is very important when studying the effects of chronic exposures.

B. The Human Experience

Some late effects studied in the past are the following:

1. Cancer and leukemia in U.S. radiologists in the 1920s to 1930s.
2. Thyroid tumors in children treated with x-rays for enlargement of the thymus.
3. Cancer and leukemia in British and German patients treated with x-rays for ankylosing spondylitis (1930s).

TABLE 10.6
Late Effects in Sublethal Exposures

Dose (rem)	(Sv)	Tissues	Effects
100	(1.0)	Bone marrow	Leukemia
100	(1.0)	Lungs	Neoplasia
100	(1.0)	Breast	Neoplasia
50–100	(0.5–1.0)	Fetus	Microcephaly
50	(0.5)	Skin	Chromosome aberrations
50	(0.5)	Gonads	Temporary infertility
5	(0.05)	Leukocytes	Chromosome aberrations
2	(0.02)	Fetus	Leukemia, tumors

4. Anemia, leukemia, and tumors in radium-dial painters (1930s).
5. Leukemia and tumors in Japanese A-bomb survivors (1945 to present).
6. Lung cancer in uranium miners of Europe (1950s) and the United States (1970s).
7. Life shortening in U.S. radiologists.

With whole-body doses of 20 to 100 rem (0.2 to 1.0 Sv), mild radiation illness is followed by complete recovery. With doses below 20 rem (0.2 Sv), there is no illness. However, some late effects are expected in humans. Table 10.6 shows some of those effects observed in persons exposed accidentally and experimentally to the range of 2 to 100 rems (0.02 to 1.0 Sv).

C. Hypotheses for Late Effects

Several models have been proposed to assess the risks of low-level exposures and to set dose limits for radiation workers and the general public. In this section, three hypotheses are considered (Figure 10.10).

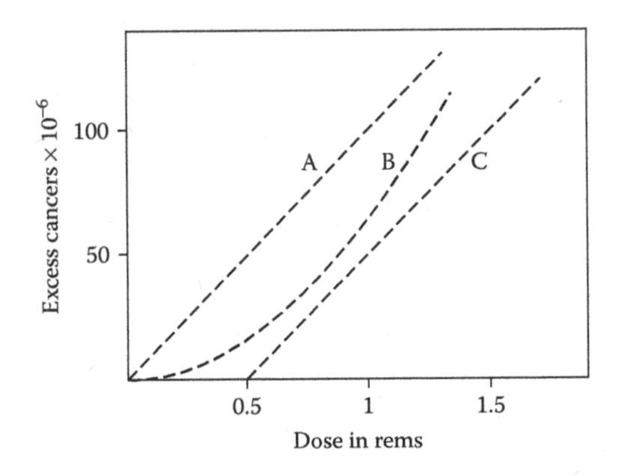

FIGURE 10.10 Three hypotheses for the late effects of radiation: A, the linear nonthreshold hypothesis (LNT); B, the linear quadratic hypothesis (LQH); and C, the threshold-linear hypothesis (TLH).

1. The linear nonthreshold hypothesis (LNT): The risk of late effects is linear with dose at all levels (curve A in Figure 10.10). The equation is

$$y = \alpha D \tag{10.3}$$

where y = risk, α = proportionality constant (slope), and D = dose.
2. The linear quadratic hypothesis (LQH): The risk of late effects is low at low doses and proportional to the square of the dose at medium and at high doses (curve B in Figure 10.10). The equation is

$$y = \alpha D + \beta D^2 \tag{10.4}$$

where α, β = components of cellular change, and D = dose.
3. The threshold linear hypothesis (TLH): There is no risk at low doses. The risk increases linearly with dose above a threshold (curve C in Figure 10.10). The equation is

$$y = \alpha D + b \tag{10.5}$$

where α = proportionality constant (slope), D = dose, and b = Y-intercept at D = 0.

D. Radiation Hormesis

1. The theory: Radiation hormesis considers that, at low levels above background, ionizing radiations may have a desirable, beneficial effect, on biological systems. Many reports of experiments with animals, plants, tissue cultures, microorganisms, and statistical data on various groups of people have shown compelling evidence not only of no injuries but also increase in growth, lower susceptibility to illnesses, lengthening of life span, and other beneficial effects. Those observations have occurred at levels of 2 to 10 times the background radiation.
2. Mechanism: Some reports suggest that neighboring cells (bystander cells), untouched by radiation, react the same way as those irradiated, possibly through intercellular communication, enhancing the adaptive response (radiation hormesis).
3. Safety standards: Although present safety standards are based on the LNT hypothesis, many well-recognized scientists oppose it. They give sound reasons to state that the LNT hypothesis exaggerates risks at low doses and that trying to reduce exposures to background levels is a waste of time and resources.

E. The Concept of Risk

1. Definitions:
   a. Risk: Exposure to loss or injury.

TABLE 10.7
Risks of Malignancies

Case/Report	Late Effect	Excess Cases/10^6 Persons/rem, per Lifetime
A-bomb survivors	All cancers	100
BEIR V	All cancers	800
NCRP	Leukemia	50
NCRP	Breast cancer	25–200
NCRP	All cancers	500

b. Radiation injury risk: Risk coefficient × radiation dose.
c. Absolute risk: Excess cases/person/y/rad. This is also expressed as excess cases/million persons/y/rad or excess cases/person/y/Sv, and excess cases/million persons/y/Sv.
d. Relative risk: Percent increase in cases/unit of radiation dose. This is also the fractional increase in cases/unit of radiation dose.

2. Comparison of risks: Empirical calculations based on previous statistical data allows comparison of risks. For example, the following events can cause loss of life expectancy by
   a. Smoking a cigarette — Loss of 10 minutes
   b. Being 20% overweight — Loss of 2.7 y
   c. Receiving 1 rem/y — Loss of 1 d
   d. Receiving 5 rem/y — Loss of 68 d

   Most radiation workers receive less than 500 mrem/y. For that reason, risk estimates are usually expressed in terms of absolute risk: number of excess cases per person per year per rem (or per Sv), or number of excess cases per person per lifetime per rem (or per Sv). Table 10.7 gives the risks of malignancies compiled from various sources. It is important to remember that these risks apply only to populations and not to individuals.
3. Absolute risks
   a. Absolute risks of fatal cancer (ICRP, 1990) after the exposure:

4.0×10^{-4}/person/y/rem (4.0×10^{-2}/person/y/Sv) for radiation workers

5.0×10^{-4}/person/y/rem (5.0×10^{-2}/person/y/Sv) for the general public

   b. Absolute risks of genetic effects after the exposure:

4×10^{-5}/person/y/rem (4×10^{-3}/person/y/Sv) for the first two generations

1.0×10^{-4}/person/y/rem (1.0×10^{-2}/person/y/Sv) for all generations

   c. Mortality due to radiation:

50 deaths/10^6 people/y/rem (0.5 deaths/10^6 people/y/Sv) for radiation workers

1–10 deaths/10^6 people/y/rem (100–1,000 deaths/10^6 people/y/Sv) for the general public

F. Life-Span Shortening

Experiments with animals have demonstrated life-span shortening directly related to dose. The aging process is a very complex one. Among the hypotheses proposed to explain aging, the following can be mentioned:

1. Genetic: Aging is programmed in the DNA's genetic clock. In cytology, apoptosis.
2. Wear and tear: The wear and tear of DNA causes cumulative damage.
3. Immune system: The age of the immune system determines the life span.
4. Free radicals: FR damage to cells is cumulative.
5. The pituitary gland: Pituitary inhibition of the thyroid gland is programmed.
6. Glucose: Glucose binding to proteins and other key molecules interferes with metabolism.
7. Overfeeding: Cells can be overwhelmed by nutrients. Laboratory animals on semistarvation diets live longer than controls.
8. Expansion of the histohematic barrier: Measurements of the distance between capillaries and parenchymal tissues show an increase with age. The density of connective tissues between capillaries and cells increases with age. The result is a reduction in tissue functions proportional to age. The expansion of the histohematic barrier may be the result of genetic and environmental factors acting on the body over a long time.

In humans, radiation life-span shortening is estimated at 2.5 to 10 d/rem (6 to 24 h/mSv), depending on the magnitude of the dose received. For low doses, the estimate is at 0.01% of a lifetime per rem, or 2.6 d/rem (0.001% of a lifetime per mSv or 6.1 h/mSv).

G. Other Late Effects

1. Cancer: Radiation-induced cancer usually affects the thyroid gland, the skeletal system, and the skin. The latent period varies from 5 to 20 y. The probability of those cancers follows the LNT hypothesis. The absolute risks of fatal cancers are given above.
2. Leukemia: Radiation-induced leukemias, myelocytic and lymphoblastic, have a latent period of 2–3 y. Their probabilities follow the linear quadratic relationship with dose.
3. Cataracts: Cataracts are the opacification of the lenses of the eyes. In humans, radiation-induced cataracts have a threshold of 60 rems (0.6 Sv) of x- or gamma radiation. The latent period lasts several years.

XIV. GENETIC EFFECTS

A. Basic Concepts

1. Chromosome aberrations: Chromosome aberrations are visible defects observed in chromosomes caused by physical, chemical, and biological agents in nature. See also lesions in DNA earlier in this chapter.
2. Mutations: Mutations are changes in genes that result in physical or physiological changes lasting at least two generations. Physical, chemical, and biological agents can cause mutations. Most mutations are deleterious. If the cell survives, the mutation will be observable in future generations.
   a. Somatic mutations: Those that occur in somatic cells. They remain with the individual. Examples are cancer and leukemia.
   b. Genetic mutations: Those that occur in germinal cells (oogonia and spermatogonia).
3. Genetic pool: Genetic pool refers to the variety of characters determined directly or indirectly by a gene. Examples are anatomical, physiological, and psychological characteristics of individuals such as physical aptitude, color and texture of the hair, the color of the eyes, behavior, etc.
4. Genetic load: Genetic load refers to the pool of deleterious genes within a species. Examples in humans are hemophilia, color blindness, and familial illnesses.
5. Genetic equilibrium: Genetic equilibrium is the constancy of the genetic load. Figure 10.11 shows that nature is constantly introducing new deleterious mutations to the pool. The figure also shows that deleterious mutations are being eliminated by the process of natural selection. The two processes are in equilibrium. Civilization tends to increase the genetic load.
6. Genetic significant dose (GSD): GSD is the gonadal radiation dose received by the public from medical and other industries divided by the population. In the United States, the GSD is estimated at 20 to 32 mrem/y (200 - 320 μSv/y), or about 7 to 11% of background radiation from natural sources.
7. Mutation doubling dose (MDD): MDD is the radiation dose that doubles the number of natural mutations. In humans, the MDD is estimated at 50 to 250 rem (0.5 to 2.5 Sv), or 169 to 847 times natural background radiation.

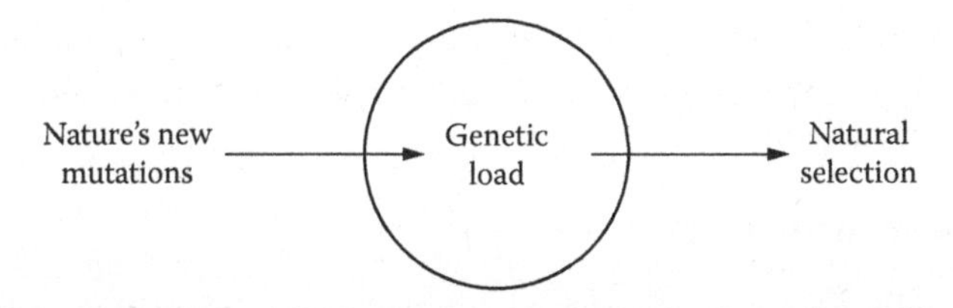

FIGURE 10.11 Within a species, the dynamic equilibrium of the genetic load, the pool of deleterious genes.

TABLE 10.8
Natural Background Radiation

Region	(mrem/y)	(mSv/y)	(rem/30 y)	(mSv/30y)[a]
Continental United States	295	(2.95)	8.85	(88.5)
Espirito Santo, Brazil	500–1000	(5–10)	15–30	(150–300)
Kerala, India	1500	(15)	45	(450)

[a] 30y is the reproductive life of a person

B. Background Radiation

All biological systems live with and tolerate background radiation well. In the United States, background radiation from natural sources is about 295 mrem/y. In other regions of the world, peoples are exposed to background radiation that can be two to five times that of the United States, apparently without any detrimental effects whatsoever. Table 10.8 compares the United States background radiation with that of two locations in other countries.

C. Mutations in *Drosophila*

H. J. Muller and followers in 1927 through 1948 demonstrated that mutations in *Drosophila melanogaster*, the fruit fly, increase linearly with radiation dose above 20 rem and that the effect was independent of dose rate.

D. The Megamouse Project

William Russell and his team of geneticists, in the 1960s and 1970s, using millions of mice, demonstrated that mutations indeed increase with radiation dose but vary directly with dose rate. They also found that, in accordance with the law of Bergonie and Tribondeau, spermatogonia are more sensitive than oocytes and that oocytes have a threshold for deleterious mutations. Of course, the threshold could also mean the oocytes can repair mutations at low doses. At higher doses, both spermatogonia and oocytes show saturation, perhaps because cell deaths prevented the observation of mutations.

XV. EFFECTS OF PRENATAL IRRADIATION

Human embryos and embryos from laboratory animals are extremely sensitive to radiation. And, the younger the developing individual, the greater the sensitivity to a given dose of radiation.

A. Experiments with Mice

Experiments with laboratory mice have permitted a description of the effects at three prenatal stages with a dose of 200 rem (2.0 Sv). The gestation period in mice lasts 20 d.

1. Preimplantation: In mice, this stage lasts 0 to 5 d. The predominant effect is prenatal death. If the embryo survives, anatomical abnormalities and neonatal death are observed.
2. Major organogenesis: This stage lasts from the 5th day to the 13th day. The predominant effects are anatomical abnormalities and neonatal death. The most frequent anatomical abnormalities observed in mice at 200 rem (2 Sv) are deficient growth, exencephaly, microcephaly, micropthalmia, limb abnormalities, snout abnormalities, and chromosome aberrations.
3. Fetal growth: This stage lasts from the 14th day to the 20th day. The most important predominant effects are physiologic abnormalities. Among them are cataracts, infertility, and life-span shortening.

B. Observations in Humans

In humans, the three prenatal stages last 10 d, 10 to 39 d, and 39 d to 9 months, respectively. Effects observed in A-bomb survivors were microcephaly, growth retardation, and mental retardation. Estimated doses received were 10 to 19 rem (100 to 190 mSv).

Other causes of anatomical abnormalities in humans include: physical: trauma; chemical: drugs such as thalidomide; and biological: the rubella (German measles) virus.

C. Recommendations

1. Diagnostic radiological procedures and NM procedures should be prescribed to pregnant women only when they are absolutely necessary and only when the benefits outweigh the risks of radiation injury to the unborn. The first trimester is the most sensitive.
2. The 10-d rule: Diagnostic radiological and NM procedures in women of childbearing age should be scheduled during the 10 d that follow the menses, which is the interval of least probability of pregnancy. A test may be required.
3. The occupational dose limit to the fetus is 50 mrem/month during the 9 months of gestation. For monitoring purposes, radiation workers must declare their pregnancy in writing.

PROBLEMS

1. In an experiment, the percentage of double-break chromosome aberrations increased with the square of the dose in sieverts. Calculate the dose for 10% aberrations.
2. The 37% dose of high-LET radiation on a cell culture is 125 rem (1.25 Sv). Calculate the dose for a 20% survival.
3. A cell culture is irradiated with ^{60}Co gamma rays. The 37% dose is 100 rem, and the extrapolated number is 2.0. What fraction would survive 50 rem?

4. If the risk is 100 excess cancers per million people per year per rem, calculate the excess cancers for a dose of 500 mrem, and express it in per person per lifetime (70 y).
5. A population of 20,000 people received 15 mrem from an accidental release of radioactivity. Assuming a risk of 100 excess cancers/million/y/rem, calculate the risk for that population during the next 70 y.

REFERENCES

Agard, E.T., Healthful radiation, *Health Phys.*, 72, 97, 1997.

BEIR V report of the National Research Council, *Health Effects of Exposure to Low Levels of Ionizing Radiation*, National Academy of Sciences, Washington, DC, 1990.

Bevalacqua, J.J., *Basic Health Physics — Problems and Solutions*, Wiley–VCH, Weinheim, Germany, 1999.

Chandra, R., *Nuclear Medicine Physics — The Basics*, 6th ed., Lippincott Williams & Wilkins, Philadelphia, PA, 2004.

Dowd, S.B. and Tilson, E.R., *Practical Radiation Protection and Applied Radiology*, 2d ed., Saunders, Philadelphia, PA, 1999.

Early, P.J. and Sodee, D.B., *Principles and Practice of Nuclear Medicine*, 2d ed., Mosby, St. Louis, MO, 1995.

Feindengen, L.E. and Pollycove, M., Biologic responses to low doses of ionizing radiation: detriment versus hormesis. Part 1. Dose responses of cells and tissues. *J. Nucl. Med.*, 42, 17N, 2001.

Goldsmith, S.J., Improving insight into radiobiology and radionuclide therapy, *J. Nucl. Med.*, 45, 1104, 2004.

LaTorre Travis, E., *Medical Radiobiology*, 2d ed., Year Book Medical Publishers, Chicago, 1989.

Marx, J., DNA repair comes into its own, *Science*, 266, 728, 1994.

Murray, R.K., Granner, D.K., Mayes, P.A., and Rodwell, V.W., *Harper's Biochemistry*, 21st ed., Appleton & Lange, Norwalk, CT, 1988.

NCRP Report 65, Management of Persons Accidentally Contaminated with Radionuclides, NCRP, Bethesda, MD, 1980.

NCRP Report 93, Ionizing Radiation Exposure of the Population of the United States, Bethesda, MD, 1987.

Noz, M.E. and Maguire, G.Q., *Radiation Protection in the Radiologic and Health Sciences*, 2d ed., Lea & Febiger, Philadelphia, PA, 1995.

Pizzarello, D.J. and Witkofski, R.L., *Medical Radiation Biology*, 2d ed., Lea & Febiger, Philadelphia, 1982.

Polycove, M., The rise and fall of the linear no-threshold theory of radiation carcinogenesis, *Nuclear News*, June 1997.

Prekeges, J.L., Radiation hormesis, *J. Nucl. Med. Technol.*, 31, 11, 2003.

Rockwell, T., What's wrong with being cautious?, *Nuclear News*, June 1997.

Saha, G.B., *Physics and Radiobiology of Nuclear Medicine*, Springer–Verlag, New York, 1993.

Schleipman, A.R. et al., Radiation disaster response: preparation and simulation experience at an academic medical center, *J. Nucl. Med. Technol.*, 32, 22, 2004.

Schull, W.J., *Effects of Atomic Radiation — A Half Century of Studies from Hiroshima and Nagasaki*, Wiley–Liss, New York, 1995.

Shani, G., *Radiation Dosimetry — Instrumentation and Methods*, 2d ed., CRC Press, Boca Raton, FL, 2000.

Shleien, B., Slaback, Jr., L.A., and Birky, B.K., *Handbook of Health Physics and Radiological Health*, 3d ed., Lippincott Williams & Wilkins, Philadelphia, PA, 1998.

Slater, R.J., *Radioisotopes in Biology*, 2d ed., Oxford University Press, Oxford, UK, 2002.

Statkiewicz-Sherer, M.A., Visconti, P.J., and Ritenour, E.R., *Radiation Protection in Medical Radiography*, 2d ed., Mosby, St. Louis, MO, 1993.

Turner, J.E., Editor, *Atoms, Radiation, and Radiation Protection*, 2d ed., John Wiley & Sons, New York, 1995.

Appendix A — Properties of Medical Radionuclides

A. NEGATRON EMITTERS

Nuclide	Half-Life	β^- E_{max} MeV (%)	Maximum Range in Soft Tissue (mm)
^{32}P	14.3 d	1.71 (100)	8.0
^{89}Sr	50.5 d	1.46 (100)	6.6
^{153}Sm	1.9 d	0.81 (44)	2.5
^{186}Re	3.8 d	1.08 (77)	4.3
^{188}Re	16.8 h	2.12 (79)	10.0
^{90}Sr	28 y	0.546 (100)	1.8
^{90}Y	64 h	2.28 (100)	12.2
^{177}Lu	6.7 d	0.497 (79)	1.5

B. GAMMA (X-RAY) EMITTERS

Nuclide	Half-Life	Photon Energies in keV (%)	Gamma Constant[a] in R/mCi-h at 1 cm
^{99m}Tc	6 h	140 (88)	0.78
^{123}I	13.1 h	159 (84)	2.2
^{111}In	2.8 d	173 (89), 247 (94)	3.21
^{133}Xe	5.3 d	81 (36), 32 (48)	0.15
^{131}I	8.05 d	364 (82)	2.2
^{125}I	60 d	35 (7), x-rays 27–32 (136)	1.41
^{67}Ga	78 h	93 (40), 184 (24), 300 (22)	1.6
^{51}Cr	27.8 d	320 (9)	0.18
^{57}Co	270 d	123 (87), 136 (11)	0.96
^{99}Mo	66 h	740 (12), 780 (4)	1.45
^{59}Fe	45 d	1100 (56), 1290 (43)	6.5
^{201}Tl	73 h	135(2), 167 (8), x-rays 69–83 (94)	0.46
^{137}Cs	30 y	662 (84)	3.3

Note: To convert R/mCi h at 1 cm into μSv/GBq h at 1 m, multiply by 27. See also Table 2.3.

C. POSITRON EMITTERS (ANNIHILATION RADIATION)

Nuclide	Half-Life	β^+E_{max} MeV (%)	β^+ Range in Soft Tissue (mm)	511 keV Photons (%)	Gamma Constant R/mCi-h at 1 cm
^{18}F	110 min	0.634 (97)	2.4	194	5.73
^{11}C	20.4 min	0.960 (99+)	5.91	200	5.91
^{13}N	10 min	1.20 (100)	5.4	200	5.91
^{15}O	2 min	1.732 (100)	8.2	200	5.91
^{68}Ga	68 min	1.9 (86)	9.1	176	6.63
^{82}Rb	75 s	3.356 (87)	15.6	192	6.1

Note: To convert R/mCi-h at 1 cm into μSv/GBq-h at 1 m, multiply by 27. See also Table 2.3.

Appendix B — Symbols and Abbreviations

A	Activity, mass number
$\tilde{A}$	Cumulative activity
ALARA	As low as reasonably achievable
α	Alpha radiation, proportionality constant
ALI	Annual limit on intake
amu	Atomic mass unit, Dalton (Da)
Å	Angstrom (10^{-10} m)
ARS	Acute radiation syndrome
BGO	Bismuth germanate
Bq	becquerel
Bkg	Background radiation
β^-	Beta (negatron)
β^+	Beta (positron)
B.C.E.	Before the common era
BM	Bone marrow
C	coulomb
c	Speed of light
c	Counts
CEA	Carcinoembryonic antigen
c/m, CPM	Counts per minute
c/s, CPS	Counts per second
cm	Centimeters
chi	χ, Greek letter
Ci	curie
CFR	Code of Federal Regulations
cGy	Centigray (rad)
CF	Correction factor
cos	Cosine
CT	Computerized tomography
CV	Coefficient of variation
D	Absorbed dose
Da	dalton, amu

DAC	Derived air concentration
D_β	Beta dose
D_γ	Gamma dose
Δ_i	Equilibrium dose constant
d	Days
DIS	Decay in storage
DISIDA	Di-isopropyl-imino-diacetic acid
DMSA	Di-mercapto-succinic acid
DPM	Disintegrations per minute
DPS	Disintegrations per second
DOT	Department of Transportation
DTPA	Diethylene-triamine-pentaacetic acid
E	Energy, effective dose
$E(\tau)$	Committed effective dose
EAE	Effective absorbed energies
e	Base of natural logarithms
$\bar{E}_\beta$	Average energy of beta particles
E_b	Binding energy
EC	Electron capture
EDTMP	Ethylene diamine tetramethylene phosphonic acid
EM	Electromagnetic radiation
E_{max}	Maximum energy of beta particles
EPA	Environmental Protection Agency
eV	Electron volt
f value	rads/roentgen
FBD	Fibrin-binding domain
FDA	Food and Drug Administration
FDG	Fluorodeoxyglucose
g	Gram; geometric factor
G value	Number of molecules changed/100 eV
γ	Gamma rays
Γ	Gamma constant
GBq	Gigabecquerel
GeV	Giga electron volt
GFR	Glomerular filtration rate
GH	Glucoheptonate
GM	Geiger–Muller
Gy	Gray
h	Hour
H	Equivalent dose
h	Planck's constant
H_d	Deep dose

HDP	Hydroxymethylene diphosphonate
HEDP	Hydroxyethyledene phosphonic acid
HMPAO	Hydroxy-methyl-propylene-amine-oxime
H_s	Shallow dose
HSA	Human serum albumin
$H_T(\tau)$	Committed equivalent dose
$h\nu$	Photon
$h\nu'$	Deflected photon
I_t	Transmitted intensity
I_o	Original intensity
IC	Internal conversion
ICRP	International Commission on Radiation Protection
ICRU	International Commission on Radiation Units and Measurements
IND	Investigational new drug
IP	Intraperitoneal administration
IT	Isomeric transition
IV	Intravenous administration
J	Joule
JCAHO	Joint Commission on Accreditation of Health Organizations
k	Kilo; pair production
keV	Kilo-electron-volt
l	Liter
λ, λ_p	Decay constant
λ_b	Biological removal constant
λ_e	Effective removal constant
LD_{50}	Lethal dose 50%
$LD_{50/30}$	Lethal dose 50% within 30 days
LD	Lens dose
LET	Linear energy transfer
LLI	Lower large intestine
ln	Natural logarithm
log	Decimal logarithm
LSO	Lutetium oxyorthosilicate
m	Meter, mass, metastable
mm	Millimeter
MBq	Megabecquerel
MAA	Macroaggregated albumin
MCA	Multichannel analyzer
mCi	Millicurie
MDP	Methylene-di-phosphonate
MeV	Mega-electron-volt
mg	Milligram

MIBI	Methoxy-iso-butyl-isonitrile
min	Minutes
MIRD	Medical Internal Radiation Dose Committee
μg	Microgram
ml	Milliliter
μm	Micrometer
MAb, MoAb	Monoclonal antibody
mR	Milliroentgens
mR/h	Milliroentgens per hour
mrem	Millirems
μSv	Microsievert
mSv	Millisievert
N	Neutron number; number of atoms
n	Number
n	Neutron
NaI(Tl)	Sodium iodide activated with thallium
NBS	National Bureau of Standards
nCi	Nanocurie
NCRP	National Council on Radiation Protection and Measurement
NDA	New drug application
NM	Nuclear medicine
NMD	Nuclear physician
NMP, NPh	Nuclear pharmacist
NMT	Nuclear medicine technologist
ν	Neutrino
NP-59	Beta-iodo-methyl 19-norcholesterol
$\bar{\nu}$	Antineutrino
NRC	Nuclear Regulatory Commission
O	Oxygen
p	Proton
pCi	Picocurie
PET	Positron emission tomography
pH	Power hydrogen
PMT	Photomultiplier tube
Q	Quantity of electrical charge, quality factor
QA	Quality assurance
QMP	Quality management program
R	roentgen; count rate
r	Count rate; radius
rad	Radiation absorbed dose
R_b	Count rate of background
R_g	Gross count rate

RBC	Red blood cells
rem	Roentgen equivalent man
RES	Reticuloendothelial system
ρ	Density
RF	Reliability factor
RP	Radiopharmaceutical
RSC	Radiation safety committee
RSO	Radiation safety officer
RSP	Radiation safety program
S	Specific ionization
s, sec	Second
s	Sample
σ	Standard deviation; Compton effect
σ_s	Sample standard deviation
σ_R	Standard deviation of count rate
SCA	Single-channel analyzer
SI	Small intestine
S.I.	International System of Units
SPECT	Single-photon emission computerized tomography
Σ	Sum of
Sv	Sievert
T	Kinetic energy
t	Time, elapsed time
τ	Mean life, relative error, photoelectric effect
T_b	Biological half-time
T_e	Effective half-life
t_b	Counting time of background
TC	Time constant
t_g	Gross counting time
TLD	Thermoluminescence dosimetry
T_2O	Tritiated water
ULI	Upper large intestine
USP	U.S. Pharmacopeia
V	Volt
W	Watt
W	Ionization potential
WB	Whole-body
WBC	White blood cells
wk	Weeks
W_R	Radiation weighting factor
W_T	Tissue weighting factor
X	Exposure, x-rays

x	Unknown, shield thickness
$\bar{x}$	Arithmetic mean
X_i	Individual observation
χ^2	Chi-squared
y	Year
Z	Atomic number

Appendix C — Interconversion of Units

The classic units appear on the first column. The S.I. units appear on the second column. To convert classic units into S.I. units, multiply the units in the first column by the factor in the third column. To reverse the process, divide the S.I. units by the same factor.

To Convert	Into	Multiply by
	A. Radioactivity	
μCi	kBq	37
mCi	MBq	37
Ci	GBq	37
	B. Exposure Rate[a]	
mR/h	μSv/h	10
R/h	mSv/h	10
	C. Absorbed Dose	
mrad	μGy	10
rad	mGy	10
	D. Equivalent Dose	
mrem	μSv	10
rem	mSv	10
	E. Dose Rate	
mrem/h	μSv/h	10
rem/h	mSv/h	10
	F. Dosimetry[a]	
rad/mCi	μSv/MBq	270
rad/mCi	mSv/MBq	0.27
rad/μCi-h	mSv/kBq-h	0.27
	G. Gamma Constant[b]	
R/mCi-h at 1 cm	μSv/GBq-h at 1 m	27

[a] μSv/h, mSv/h, for negatrons, positrons, gamma, and x-rays.

[b] Gamma constant is the intensity or flux of photons/cm^2 at 1 cm or at 1 m from the source.

Appendix D — Answers to Problems

CHAPTER 1

1. Express the elapsed time and the half-life in the same time units. Use Equation 1.3.
   Answer: 278.6 MBq/ml.
2. First calculate decay using Equation 1.3; then use a proportion to determine the volume needed.
   Answer: 1.17 ml.
3. Use Equation 1.3 first, and then subtract the excretion.
   Answer: 2.65 GBq.
4. The unknown is the original activity (A_0). Use Equation 1.3 and solve for A_0.
   Answer: 1.53 GBq.
5. Rate of decay is the same as decay constant.
   Answers: Rate of ^{99}Mo: 0.0105 h^{-1} or 1.05% h^{-1}.
   Rate of ^{99m}Tc: 0.1155 h^{-1} or 11.55% h^{-1}.
6. Use Equation 1.3, and take the reciprocal of e^{-x}, apply natural logarithms to both sides.
   Answer: 4.42 h or 4 h and 25 min.
7. Use Equation 1.3, follow procedure in Problem 6.
   Answer: 1.93 h or 1 h and 56 min or at 7:56 a.m.
8. Similar to Problem 6.
   Answer: 12.8 h or 12 h and 49 min.
9. Use Equation 1.1, enter half-life in seconds, then divide by the definition of microcurie.
   Answer: 0.89 μCi or 32.9 kBq.
10. Use Equation 1.3.
    Answer: 128 kBq or 3.46 μCi.

CHAPTER 2

1. Soft tissues have the same absorption coefficients as water. Divide by the density of water: 1000 mg/cm^3.
   Answer: 0.8 cm or 8 mm.

2. Similar to problem 1.
   Answer: 12.2 mm.
3. The specific gamma constant of ^{226}Ra is 222.8 µSv/GBq-h at 1 m. Use a proportion and the inverse-square law.
   Answer: 4.95 µSv/h at 30 cm.
4. Table 2.1 gives a w_R of 10 for 50-keV neutrons and 1 for gamma rays. Multiply each dose times its factor and add the products.
   Answer: 1,020 mSv or 1.02 Sv.
5. Table 2.4 gives the following specific gamma constants: ^{123}I: 44.0; ^{131}I: 61.3; ^{111}In: 86.7; and ^{99m}Tc: 21.1, all in µSv/GBq-h at 1 m.
6. Similar to the previous question.
   Answers: ^{18}F: 154.7; ^{13}N: 159.6; ^{11}C: 159.6; and ^{82}Rb: 164.7, all in µSv/GBq-h at 1 m.
7. The $\bar{E}_\beta$ is about 1/3 of the E_{max}. Find the E_{max} in Table 1.4 and divide by 3.
   Answers: ^{32}P: 570 keV, ^{89}Sr: 497 keV; ^{186}Re: 359 keV; and ^{90}Y: 795 keV.
8. Similar to the previous question; use Table 1.5.
   Answers:^{18}F: 211 keV; ^{13}N: 400 keV; ^{11}C: 320 keV; and ^{82}Rb: 1.12 MeV.
9. Use the gamma constant, a proportion, and the inverse square law.
   Answer: 34.4 µSv/h.
10. Similar to the previous question. Convert inches to centimeters. Apply the inverse square law.
    Answer: 1.2 mSv/h.

CHAPTER 3

1. Use Equation 1.3 and solve for time.
   Answer: 4.96 h, or 4 h and 58 min.
2. Decay factor for five half-lives is $e^{-0.693 \times 5} = 0.03125$, or 3.13% (answer).
3. Apply the inverse square law.
   Answer: 25.6 cm.
4. Doubling the distance decreases the exposure by a factor of 4, and doubling the time increases it by a factor of 2.
   Answer: 90 µSv.
5. Three HVLs would reduce it to 20 µSv/h. The HVL for ^{99}Mo is 7 mm of lead (Table 6.2). Therefore, 3×7 mm = 21 mm or 2.1 cm of Pb (answer). Alternatively, Equation 6.4 may be used.
6. Similar to Problem 2.
   Answer: 3.13%.
7. Divide what you want by (mCi) what you have (mCi/ml).
   Answer: 1.43 ml.
8. The elapsed time is 26 h. Express the half-life in hours. Use Equation 1.3.
   Answer: 367 MBq/ml.
9. Calculate concentration at noon and then divide into 50 MBq.
   Answer: 0.65 ml.

10. Problem of decay. Express the elapsed time in days.
    Answer: 248.7 MBq/ml.

CHAPTER 4

1. Obtain the two count rates, apply Equation 4.3, and subtract bkg.
   Answer: 592 ± 12 c/m.
2. Use Equation 4.1 and Equation 4.2.
   Answer: 2,641± 28 c/m.
3. CV = $\sigma_s \times$ 100/mean, and Equation 4.4 gives the standard error.
   Answers: CV = 1.06% and $\sigma_{\bar{x}} = \pm$ 12.4 c/m.
4. Answers: RF = 28/2,641$^{1/2}$ = 0.54 (acceptable at the 96% confidence range); Use Equation 4.7 to obtain χ^2 = 1.17 (acceptable). The instrument is operating well.
5. Acceptable for five observations: mean ± 1.64σ_s or 2,595 – 2,687 c/m.
   Answer: None can be rejected.
6. Use Equation 4.5 and Table 4.4. The relative error is 3.5 standard deviations and therefore is unacceptable.
   Answer: The camera is contaminated.
7. Use Equation 4.1 and 4.2.
   Answers: Mean ± σ_s = 8.1 ± 1.8 μg/dl; 95% range: 4.5 to 11.7 μg/dl.
8. Acceptable for ten observations: mean ± 1.97σ_s or 4.55 to 11.65 μg/dl.
   Answer: None can be rejected.
9. Use the MDA formula:
   Answer: 2.1×10^{-5} μCi.
10. Use Equation 4.5 and Table 4.6. The relative error is 1.9 standard deviations, which is acceptable. The detector is operating well.

CHAPTER 5

1. Apply the decay Equation 1.3 and a proportion.
   Answer: 0.46 ml.
2. Use the decay equation.
   Answer: 91.4 MBq/ml.
3. Use the decay equation.
   Answer: 227 MBq.
4. Decay the total amount and then subtract the excreted part.
   Answer: 0.32 GBq.
5. Use $V_1 \times C_1 = V_2 \times C_2$ formula. Then, subtract V_1 from V_2.
   Answer: 3.0 ml of saline.
6. Calculate decay and use a proportion.
   Answer: 0.65 ml.
7. Use the decay equation.
   Answer: Each capsule contains 0.057 MBq or 1.54 μCi of ^{123}I.

8. Correct for 25-h decay. ^{99}Mo half-life is 66 h.
   Answer: 16.9 GBq.
9. For 10% use the following: $0.1 = e^{-0.693t}$, where t is the elapsed time in half-lives. Similar equations are used for 0.01 (1%) and 0.001 (0.1%).
   Answers: 10%, 3.3 half-lives; 1%, 6.6 half lives; and 0.1%, 9.9 half-lives.
10. Use the decay equation.
    Answer: 13.1 h.

CHAPTER 6

1. Use the inverse square law (Equation 6.3).
   Answer: 65.2 cm.
2. Use the shielding equation (Equation 6.4).
   Answer: 3.44 cm of lead.
3. Time was reduced to one-half. Solution: 180 µSv/2 = 90 µSv (answer).
4. Use shielding equation (see Problem 2).
   Answer: 2.92 cm of lead.
5. Use Equation 6.4.
   Answer: 0.325 or 32.5%.
6. One mm of lead is equal to 4 HVLs.
   Answer: 6.25%.
7. Answer: No reason to panic. 750 µSv/h is well below the 1,000 µSv/h limit on the surface of category III packages shipped by passenger airlines.
8. Use a proportion and the inverse square law formula.
   Answer: 1,243 µSv/h.
9. Similar to Problem 8.
   Answer: 3.3 µSv/h.
10. Multiply the gamma constant times 2 and divide by 4.
    Answer: 77.4 µSv/h.

CHAPTER 7

1. Dose limits are given in Chapter 3.
   Answer: 15 rem/y or 150 mSv/y.
2. Answer: 50 rem/y or 500 mSv/y.
3. Answer: at 70 µm.
4. Answer: 50 mrem/month or 500 µSv/month after pregnancy is declared.
5. Answer: No. 1 mrem is (10 µSv).
6. Answer: 50 rem/y or 500 mSv/y.
7. Answer: 5 rem/y or 50 mSv/y.
8. Answers from Table 2.4:
   ^{99}Mo, 1.47 R/mCi-h at 1 cm or 39.7 µSv/GBq-h at 1 m.
   ^{99m}Tc, 0.78 R/mCi-h at 1 cm or 21.1 µSv/GB-h at 1 m.

9. Answer: 10 mrem/y of continuous exposure (100 μSv/y).
10. Answer: 10 mrem/y represents a risk of 1 excess cancer/10,000 persons.

CHAPTER 8

1. Use the decay equation.
   Answer: 8.49 GBq.
2. Divide by 10 to obtain the initial concentration. Then calculate decay for 3 h.
   Answer: 0.92 GBq/ml.
3. Answer: Category III. Limit on surface: 100 mR/h (1,000 μSv/h) for passenger airline shipping.
4. Decay and proportion.
   Answer: 2.22 ml.
5. Decay for 68 h.
   Answer: 13.7 GBq.
6. Use the equation 5.1.
   Answer: 3.86 h or 3h and 52 min or at 11:52 AM.
7. 50 nCi = 0.05 μCi. Use Table 5.4.
   Answer: Yes, it can be used within 10 h and 30 min.
8. Decay and proportion.
   Answer: 3.37 ml.
9. Decay and proportion.
   Answer: 0.7 ml
10. Use the decay equation.
    Answer: 2.04 GBq.

CHAPTER 9

1. Take 30% of 10 μCi and use Equations 9.5 and 9.7.
   Answer: 16 rads (160 mGy).
2. Similar to Problem 1.
   Answer: 1.88 rads (18.8 mGy).
3. Multiply by 1.7.
   Answer: 25.5 rem = 255 mSv = 0.255 Sv.
4. Use Equations 9.5 and 9.7.
   Answer: 0.0675 rad (0.675 mGy)
5. Similar to Problem 4.
   Answer: 2.08 rads (20.8 mGy).
6. Similarly, the answer is 0.658 rad (6.58 mGy).
7. Answer: 0.0012 rad = 1.2 mrad (12 μSv).
8. Use a proportion.
   Answer: 150 mrad (1.5 mGy).

9. Calculate the dose from each and add the three doses to obtain: 802 mrad (8.02 mGy) (answer).
10. Use a proportion.
    Answer: 7.92 rad (79.2 mGy).

CHAPTER 10

1. Use 10% = D^2.
   Answer: 3.16 Sv.
2. Use Equation 10.1.
   Answer: 201 rems (2.01 Sv).
3. Use Equation 10.2.
   Answer: 0.845 or 84.5%.
4. Divide by 2, divide by onc million, and multiply by 70.
   Answer: 3.5×10^{-3} cancers per person per 70 y.
5. Similar to Problem 4.
   Answer: 2.1 cancers per 20,000 persons per 70 y.

Index

A

Abbreviations, 205–210
A-bomb survivors, 193, 195, 199
Absolute standardization, 31
Absorbed dose, 32
Absorbed fraction, MIRD method, 157
Acetyl coenzyme A, 173, 174
ACR, *see* American College of Radiology
Actinomycin, 188
Acute lymphoblastic leukemias, 120
Acute radiation syndrome (ARS), 49, 178, 189
Adenosine diphosphate (ADP), 173
Adenosine triphosphate (ATP) synthases, 173
ADP, *see* Adenosine diphosphate
Adriamycin, 188
Aerobic glycolysis, 173
Aerosols, 135
Aging, 196
ALARA, 52–52
  objective, 92
  policy, 47, 103
  radiobiology and, 171
Alarm monitors, 126, 127
ALI, *see* Annual limit on intake
Alpha decay, 10
Alpha emitters, 113
Alpha interactions
  range, 20
  specific ionization, 20
  trajectory, 19
AMA, *see* American Medical Association
American College of Radiology (ACR), 45
American Medical Association (AMA), 45
American Nuclear Society (ANS), 45
Anaerobic glycolysis, 173
Animal care, regulations of, 172
Annihilation radiation, 13, 21, 24, 116
Annual limit on intake (ALI), 50, 136, 140, 163
ANS, *see* American Nuclear Society
Antineutrino, 12
ARS, *see* Acute radiation syndrome
Artificial alphas, 11
Artificial radioactivity, discovery of, 2
Atom, 1, 7
Atomic particles, basic, 7
Atomic structure, 6
ATP synthases, *see* Adenosine triphosphate synthases
Attenuation factors, estimation of, 109
Avogadro's number, 2, 17

B

Background radiation, 72, 198
Bacteria, 172
Becquerel, Henri, 41
Bergonie and Tribondeau, law of, 186, 191, 198
Beta interactions
  annihilation radiation, 21
  backscatter, 21
  bremsstrahlung, 21
  range, 20
  trajectory, 20
Beta particles, range of, 35
BGO, *see* Bismuth germanate
Big Bang, 105
Biohazards, 134
Biological half-lives, 166, 167
Biological models
  highly diffusible radionuclides, 164
  high-organ-uptake radionuclides, 165
Biological system
  conditions, 178
  experimental design, 177
  method of observation, 178
  systems studies, 177
Bismuth germanate (BGO), 69
Black holes, 3
Bleepers, 148
Bleomycin, 188
Blood volume test, 84
Blunders, 70
Bohr, Niels, 3
Bone marrow syndrome, 190
Bone metastases, palliation of pain in, 161
Bragg curve, 20
Braking radiation, 21
Bremsstrahlung, 21
Byproduct materials, 46

C

D

E

Electron(s), 2
capture (EC), 14, 15
-hole, 145
transport chain, 174
traps, 143
Electronic collimation, 69
EM radiations, *see* Electromagnetic radiations
Energy
currency, cell metabolism, 173
flow
law of, 5
living organisms, 172
gamma ray interactions as function of, 25
MKS system, 6
recoil, 11
Entropy, law of, 5
Environmental Protection Agency (EPA), 42, 43, 136, 150
EPA, *see* Environmental Protection Agency
Equation, high-LET curve, 185
Equilibrium dose constants, MIRD method, 157
Equivalent dose, 32
Error(s)
random, 70
relative, 74, 75, 76
systematic, 70
Ethylene diamine tetramethylene phosphonic acid (EDTMP), 120
Excretion function, 164
Exposure(s)
effect of shielding, 106
external, 139
occupational, 136, 140
rate constant, 37, 38
time of, 104
whole-body, 139, 189, 190

F

FAD, *see* Flavine adenine dinucleotide
FAO, *see* United Nations Food and Agricultural Organization
FDA, *see* Food and Drug Administration
FDG, *see* Fluorodeoxyglucose
Fermi, Enrico, 4
Fever of unknown origin (FUO), 88–89
Film
badge dosimetry, 141
badge services, advantages of, 145
calibration curve, 144
processing, 143
Flavine adenine dinucleotide (FAD), 174
Fluorine-18 decay, 13
Fluorodeoxyglucose (FDG), 115
Flux, 31
Food and Drug Administration (FDA), 42, 43
Forces of nature, 5
Free radicals (FRs), 179, 181
damage to cells, 196
scavengers, 188
Frozen energy, matter as, 4
FRs, *see* Free radicals
FUO, *see* Fever of unknown origin
f value, 35

G

Gamma constant, 37, 38
Gamma decay, 15
Gamma emitters, 15, 31, 116, 203
Gamma fraction, 31
Gamma ray
attenuation, 25
interactions
Compton effect, 22
general considerations, 21
internal conversion, 24
pair production, 23
photoelectric effect, 21
spectrometers, multichannel, 59
Gas detectors, 58, 59
components, 59
diagram of, 60
ions collected and voltage, 59
properties of, 65
responses, 60
uses of, 65
Gated SPECT, 68
Gaussian distribution, 71
Geiger–Muller (GM) survey meters, 57, 58, 123
calibration of, 62, 126
design, 61
disadvantage, 62
error of detection, 61
gases, 61
scales, 61
time constant, 62
wall thickness, 61
Geissler, Henrich, 2
General licenses, 48
General public dose limits, 51
Genes, 183
Genetic pool, 197
Genetic significant dose (GSD), 197
Germinal cells, 174
GI syndrome, 190
GM survey meters, *see* Geiger–Muller survey meters

Green plants, 172
GSD, *see* Genetic significant dose
Guidelines for radiation protection, 41–55
national and international agencies, 41–45
big picture, 41–42
Department of Transportation, 44–45
Environmental Protection Agency, 43
Food and Drug Administration, 43–44
International Commission on Radiation Protection, 42–43
International Commission on Radiation Units and Measurements, 43
Joint Commission on Accreditation of Health Organizations, 45
National Council on Radiation Protection and Measurement, 42
Nuclear Regulatory Commission, 43
other consulting organizations, 45
other concepts in dosimetry, 49–51
annual limit on intake, 50
committed effective dose, 49
committed equivalent dose, 49
deep dose, 50
derived air concentrations, 50
lens dose, 51
shallow dose, 50
problems, 54
radiation safety and the law, 46–48
ALARA policy, 47
concept of risk, 47
licensing, 48
method, 47–48
objective, 46
philosophy, 46
radiation safety practice, 52–54
ALARA program, 52–53
quality management program, 52
radiation safety committee, 52
radiation safety officer, 52
radiation safety program, 52
radiation warning signs, 53–54
rationale, 41
recommended dose limits, 51
comments, 51
general public dose limits, 51
occupational dose limits, 51
types of radiation effects, 48–49
acute and chronic exposures, 48
deterministic effects, 48–49
stochastic effects, 49

H

Half-life, decay and, 8
Half-value layer (HVL), 107, 109
H & D curve, 144
Health Physics Society (HPS), 45
High-level wastes (HLW), 132
Histones, 183
HIV, *see* Human immunodeficiency virus
HLW, *see* High-level wastes
Hot areas, 83
Hot lab, 85, 87, 125, 129
HPS, *see* Health Physics Society
Human cell, composition of, 182
Human immunodeficiency virus (HIV), 112, 172
HVL, *see* Half-value layer
Hybrid scanner, 70
Hyperthyroidism, 12, 117

I

IAEA, *see* International Atomic Energy Agency
ICRP, *see* International Commission on Radiation Protection
ICRU, *see* International Commission on Radiation Units and Measurements
Image density, 143
Imaging
planar, 68
procedures
radionuclides, 86
technetium-99m, 85
rooms, 84
Incident reports, 150
IND, *see* Investigational new drug
Indium-111 decays, 16
Internal contamination
accidental injection, 112
ingestion, 110
inhalation, 110
percutaneous absorption, 111
Internal conversion, 24
Internal dosimetry and bioassays, 153–169
bioassay of radioactivity, 162–166
airborne medical radionuclides, 163
bioassays of iodine-131, 163–164
biological models, 164–166
definitions, 162–163
requirements, 163
biological half-times, 166
historical review, 153–160
general considerations, 153–154
ICRP method, 154–156
methods, 154
MIRD method, 156–159
RADAR web site, 159–160

internal doses from radiopharmaceuticals, 160–162
diagnostic RPs, 160–162
package inserts, 160
problems, 167
rationale, 153
International Atomic Energy Agency (IAEA), 42, 43, 45
International Commission on Radiation Protection (ICRP), 42, 154
International Commission on Radiation Units and Measurements (ICRU), 42, 43
Intrinsic peak efficiency, gamma emitter, 31
Inverse square law, 32, 105
Investigational new drug (IND), 43–44
Iodine-125, 120
Iodine-131, 120, 163
Ionization chambers, 63, 126, 127
Irradiation
effects, theories of, 179
prenatal, 198
Isomeric transition (IT), 15
Isotopes, 8
IT, *see* Isomeric transition

J

JCAHO, *see* Joint Commission on Accreditation of Health Organizations
JNM, see *Journal of Nuclear Medicine*
Joint Commission on Accreditation of Health Organizations (JCAHO), 45
Joliot, Frederick, 2
Journal of Nuclear Medicine (JNM), 156

K

Krebs cycle, 174
Kupffer cells, 176

L

Laboratory
rules, 96, 112–113
surveys, 98
Lavoisier, Antoine, 2
Law of Bergonie and Tribondeau, 186, 191, 198
Law of conservation of mass or energy, 5
Law of energy flow, 5
Law of entropy, 5
Laws of thermodynamics, 4
Lead, properties of, 24
Lens dose, 51
LET, *see* Linear energy transfer
Leukemia, 192, 193
acute lymphoblastic, 120
radiation-induced, 196
Leukocyte count, 190
Licensing, 48
Life-span shortening, 196
Linear accelerator, invention of, 2
Linear attenuation coefficient, 107
Linear energy transfer (LET), 35, 187
Linear nonthreshold hypothesis (LNT), 194
Linear quadratic hypothesis (LQH), 194
Liquid wastes, 133, 135
Living organisms
defense mechanisms, 175
properties of, 171–172
LLW, *see* Low-level wastes
LNT, *see* Linear nonthreshold hypothesis
Low-level wastes (LLW), 133
LQH, *see* Linear quadratic hypothesis
LSO crystal detectors, *see* Lutetium oxyorthosilicate crystal detectors
Lukewarm areas, 82
Lutetium oxyorthosilicate (LSO) crystal detectors, 69
Lymphocyte count, 190

M

MAb, *see* Monoclonal antibody
Magnetic quantum number, 3
Magnetic resonance imaging (MRI), 82
Major spills, 98
Malignancies, risk of, 195
Marinelli equations, 154, 155
Mass, 5
attenuation coefficient, 107
–energy equivalence, 6
Matter, nature of, 1
MCA, *see* Multichannel analyzer
MDA, *see* Minimum detectable activity
MDD, *see* Mutation doubling dose
Mean absorbed doses, 158
Medical Internal Radiation Dose (MIRD) Committee, 156
assumptions, 156
equations, 157
internal doses, 159
Medical radionuclides
half-lives of, 9
half-value layers of, 109
properties of, 203–204
gamma emitters, 203

negatron emitters, 203
positron emitters, 204
Megamouse project, 198
Meiosis, 174
Methotrexate, 188
Microscopic autoradiography, 184
Minimum detectable activity (MDA), 75
MIRD Committee, *see* Medical Internal Radiation Dose Committee
Mitosis, 174, 175
MKS system, 6, 32
Molecular medicine, 86
Monoclonal antibody (MAb), 88, 162
MRI, *see* Magnetic resonance imaging
Multichannel analyzer (MCA), 59, 67
Mutation doubling dose (MDD), 197
Mutations, 197

N

NAD, *see* Nicotinamide dinucleotide
NAS, *see* National Academy of Sciences
NAS-BEIR, *see* National Academy of Sciences–Biological Effects of Ionizing Radiation
National Academy of Sciences (NAS), 42
National Academy of Sciences–Biological Effects of Ionizing Radiation (NAS-BEIR), 45
National Bureau of Standards (NBS), 45
National Certification Board Exam, 93
National Council on Radiation Protection and Measurement (NCRP), 42
National Institutes of Health (NIH), 45, 172
National Science Foundation (NSF), 42, 45, 172
National Voluntary Laboratory Accreditation Program (NVLAP), 141
Nature, forces of, 5
NBS, *see* National Bureau of Standards
NCRP, *see* National Council on Radiation Protection and Measurement
Negatron
decay, 11
emitters, 12, 114, 203
Neutron(s), 116
–boron interaction, 117
capture, 4
NHL, *see* Non-Hodgkins lymphoma
Nicotinamide dinucleotide (NAD), 174
NIH, *see* National Institutes of Health
NM, *see* Nuclear medicine
NMDs, *see* Nuclear physicians
NMTs, *see* Nuclear medicine technologists
Non-Hodgkins lymphoma (NHL), 12, 114, 120
Nonimaging room, 82, 83, 125
Nonrestricted areas, NM department, 82
Nonthreshold, linear dose–effect relationship, 46
Normal distribution
background radiation, 72
coefficient of variation, 73
meaning of σ_s, 72
practical rules, 72
ranges of confidence, 71
rejection of data, 74
reliability, 73
sample, 71
standard deviation of the mean, 73
total counts collected, 73
NRC, *see* Nuclear Regulatory Commission
NSF, *see* National Science Foundation
Nuclear medicine (NM), 1, 41
gamma emitters in, 16
negatron emitters in, 12
packages, 44
positron emitters in, 14
technologists (NMTs), 48, 123, 139
wastes, 133
Nuclear medicine department, radiation safety in, 81–101
ALARA program, 92–93
description of areas, 83–86
control room, 84
imaging rooms, 84–85
nonimaging procedures room, 83–84
radiopharmacy, 85–86
waiting room and reception, 83
design of NM department, 82–83
cold areas, 82
hot areas, 83
lukewarm areas, 82
warm areas, 83
map, 128
molecular medicine, 86–89
practice of radiation safety, 93–98
authorized users, 93
dose calibrators, 95–96
inspections, 94
laboratory rules, 96
laboratory surveys, 98
personnel exposures, 93
radiation emergencies, 98
radioactive waste disposal, 96–97
radionuclide therapy, 98
radiopharmaceuticals, 95
reception of radioactive packages, 94
record keeping, 93–94
sealed sources, 98
training of personnel, 93
use of radioactive materials, 96

problems, 99–100
quality management program, 91–92
definition, 91
misadministrations, 92
recordable events, 92
reportable events, 92
radiation safety committee, 90
radiation safety officer, 90–91
radiation safety program, 89–90
contents, 90
general considerations, 89–90
radioactive materials license, 91
radioactive spills in, 130
rationale, 81
workhorses of, 63
Nuclear physicians (NMDs), 48
Nuclear Regulatory Commission (NRC), 41, 43
Nucleus, stability of, 8
Nuclide, 8, 134
NVLAP, *see* National Voluntary Laboratory Accreditation Program

O

Occupational dose limits, 51
Occupational exposures, 136, 140
Occupational Safety and Health Administration (OSHA), 45
OER, *see* Oxygen enhancement ratio
Optically stimulated luminescence (OSL), 148
Orbitals, 4
Organ(s)
effective radius of, 154
masses of standard man, 155
OSHA, *see* Occupational Safety and Health Administration
OSL, *see* Optically stimulated luminescence
OSL dosimetry, 148, 149
Osteomyelitis, 88
Overkill effect, 188
Oxidases, 173
Oxidative decarboxylation, 174
Oxygen enhancement ratio (OER), 187

P

Packed cell volume (PCV), 84, 190
Particle interactions, 19
Pauli, Wolfgang, 4
PCR, *see* Polymerase chain reaction
PCV, *see* Packed cell volume
Personal alarm monitors, 148
Personnel exposures, monitoring of, 139–152
monitoring methods, 141–149
acceptable methods, 141
film badge dosimetry, 141–145
OSL dosimetry, 148–149
personal alarm monitors, 148
pocket dosimeters, 146–148
thermoluminescence dosimetry, 145–146
monitoring of occupational exposures, 140
dose limits, 140
requirements, 140
problems, 151
rationale, 139
records of personnel dosimetry, 149
committed dose, 149
other records, 149
personnel doses, 149
previous records, 149
reminder of dose limits, 140–141
nonoccupational dose limits, 140–141
occupational dose limits, 140
reportable events, 150
EPA, 150
files, 150
incidents, 150
reports to individuals, 150
reports, 149–150
incident reports, 150
lost or stolen radioactive sources, 149
PET, *see* Positron emission tomography
PET/CT scanner, 57, 70, 93
Phosphorus-32, 12, 119
Phosphorylases, 173
Photoelectric effect, 21, 22
Photomultiplier tube (PMT), 66, 145
Photons, dual nature of, 17
Photosynthesis, 172
Pituitary gland, 196
Planar imaging, 68
Plank, Max, 3
Plank's constant, 17
PLD, *see* Potentially lethal damage
PMT, *see* Photomultiplier tube
Pocket dosimeters
advantage, 64, 148
applications, 64
description, 146
design, 64
disadvantages, 148
operation, 64
Poisson distribution, 70
Poliomyelitis, 172
Polonium
alpha particles, Bragg curve of, 20

decay, 11
discovery of, 2
Polymerase chain reaction (PCR), 184
Portable ionization chambers, 63
Positron, 2
decay, 13
emitters, 13, 15, 115, 204
Positron emission tomography (PET), 15, 67–68
imaging
agents, 112
metabolic tracers, 68
PET scanner, 69
radiopharmaceuticals for, 69
Potentially lethal damage (PLD), 186, 187
Prenatal irradiation, 198
Principles of radiation physics, 1–27
atomic structure and radioactivity, 6–19
basic structure, 6–7
electromagnetic radiations, 16–19
modes of radioactive decay, 10–16
nuclear stability, 7–8
radioactive decay, 8–10
brief history of radiation science, 1–4
atoms and molecules, 2
nature of matter, 1
quantum physics, 3–4
radiation physics, 4
relativity, 3
x-rays and natural radioactivity, 2
gamma ray interactions, 21–24
Compton effect, 22
general considerations, 21
internal conversion, 24
pair production, 23–24
photoelectric effect, 21–22
gamma ray interactions with lead and water, 24–26
gamma ray attenuation, 25
lead, 25–26
properties of lead, 24
properties of water, 24–25
water or soft tissue, 26
matter and energy, 4–6
basic units, 5–6
laws of thermodynamics, 4–5
nature of matter, 4
particle interactions, 19–21
alpha interactions, 19–20
beta interactions, 20–21
general considerations, 19
problems, 26
rationale, 1
Principle of uncertainty, Heissenberg's, 4
Problems
answers to, 213–218
guidelines for radiation protection, 54
internal dosimetry and bioassays, 167
nuclear medicine department, radiation safety in, 99–100
personnel exposures, monitoring of, 151
principles of radiation physics, 26
radiation detection and measurement, 78
radiation surveys and waste disposal, 137
radiobiology, 199–200
safe handling of radioactivity, 121
units of radiation exposure and dose, 39
Protective equipment, 139
Pulmonary ventilation imaging, 133, 135
Pythagoras's hypothesis, 1

Q

QA, *see* Quality assurance
QMP, *see* Quality management program
Quality assurance (QA), 57, 76, 81
Quality management program (QMP), 52, 91
Quanta, 3
Quantum theory, 3
Quarks, 7

R

RADAR web site, 159
Radiation(s)
annihilation, 13, 21, 24, 116
background, 72, 198
braking, 21
cancer and, 192
counters, quality assurance of, 76
delayed effects of, 192
deterministic effects, 192
dispersion device (RDD), 191
dose fractionation, 189
electromagnetic, 3, 16
hormesis, theory of, 194
physics, 4
-producing devices, 46
properties of, 1
protection program (RPP), 52
stochastic effects, 192
terrestrial, 176
warning signs, 53
weighting factors, 33
Radiation detection and measurement, 57–79
fundamentals, 57–59
detection, 58
interpretation, 59
measurement, 58

principles, 57–58
radiation survey instruments, 58–59
radioactive contamination, 58
gas detectors, 59–65
basic design, 59–61
calibration of GM survey meters, 62
dose calibrators, 63–64
GM survey meters, 61–62
pocket dosimeters, 64–65
portable ionization chambers, 63
summary of gas detectors, 65
wipe-test counters, 63
imaging instrumentation, 67–70
conventional imaging, 68
merging of PET and CT, 69–70
PET imaging, 68–69
making decisions, 74–75
contamination, 75
detector performance, 74
minimum detectable activity, 75–76
problems, 78
quality assurance of radiation counters, 76–78
QA tests, 76–78
reliability, 76
rationale, 57
scintillation detectors, 65–67
associated electronics, 66–67
basic design, 65–66
statistics of counting, 70–74
normal distribution, 71–74
statistical distributions, 70–71
types of errors, 70
Radiation effects
acute and chronic exposures, 48
deterministic effects, 48
stochastic effects, 49
Radiation exposure
acute exposure, 178
chronic exposure, 179
experimental levels of exposure, 179
Radiation hazards
alpha emitters, 113
gamma emitters, 116
negatron emitters, 114
neutrons, 116
positron emitters, 115
Radiation injury
biological stage, 179
direct theory, 179, 180
indirect theory, 179, 180, 181
modifiers
biological modifiers, 188
chemical modifiers, 187
dose fractionation, 189
overkill effect, 188
physical modifiers, 187
risk, 195
Radiation safety
authorized users, 93
committee (RSC), 52, 90
dose calibrators, 95
emergencies, 98
inspections, 94
laboratory rules, 96
laboratory surveys, 98
officer (RSO), 47, 48, 52, 53, 90–91
radiation surveys and, 123
TLD dosimetry and, 153
practice, 52
program (RSP), 52, 89
radioactive waste disposal, 96
radionuclide therapy, 98
radiopharmaceuticals, 95
reception of radioactive packages, 94
record keeping, 93
sealed sources, 98
training of personnel, 93
use of radioactive materials, 96
Radiation source(s)
artificial, 177
basic concepts, 29, 30
levels of radiation, 177
natural, 176
radiobiology and, 176
Radiation survey instruments
gas detectors, 58
personal exposure monitors, 59
scintillation detectors, 59
Radiation surveys and waste disposal, 123–138
accidental contamination, 130–132
decontamination, 130–132
radioactive spills, 130
release of ^{133}Xe, 132
disposal of radioactive wastes, 134–136
disposal of solid wastes, 134–135
gases, aerosols, and volatile radioiodine, 135–136
liquid wastes disposal, 135
transportation of wastes, 136
Environmental Protection Agency, 136–137
monitoring, 128–129
hot-lab housekeeping, 129
map of department, 128
method, 128–129
wipe-test monitoring, 129
occupational exposures, 136
^{131}I, 136
^{133}Xe, 136
problems, 137

radiation surveys, 123–125
alarm monitors, 126
GM survey meters, 126
ionization chambers, 126–127
methods, 125
preparation, 123–124
proper operation, 124–125
selection of survey instrument, 124
surface monitors, 127
surveying of working areas, 125
survey practices, 124
radioactive wastes, 132–134
classes of radioactive wastes, 132–133
nuclear medicine wastes, 133
radiotoxicity, 133–134
rationale, 123
survey instruments, 126–127
Radioactive contamination, 58
Radioactive decay
alpha decay, 10
decay constant, 8
electron capture, 14
gamma decay, 15
isomeric transition, 15
modes of, 10
negatron decay, 11
positron decay, 13
Radioactive gases, 133
Radioactive materials license, 91
Radioactive packages, reception of, 94
Radioactive sources, lost or stolen, 149
Radioactive waste(s)
classes of, 132
disposal, radiation safety and, 96
Radioactivity
abbreviation for, 30
absolute standardization, 31
artificial, discovery of, 2
bioassay of
airborne medical radionuclides, 163
biological models, 164
definitions, 162
iodine-131, 163
requirements, 163
quantity used, 103
relative standardization, 30
Radiobiology, 171–201
acute radiation syndrome, 189–192
bone marrow syndrome, 190
CNS syndrome, 191
GI syndrome, 190–191
radiation dispersion device, 191–192
whole-body exposure, 189
basic concepts, 171–176
cell cycle, 175
cell division, 174
cellular respiration, 173–174
defense mechanisms, 175–176
energy flow, 172
living organisms, 171
mitosis, 174–175
properties of living organisms, 171–172
DNA, 182–184
lesions, 182
role, 183–184
effects of prenatal irradiation, 198–199
experiments with mice, 198–199
observations in humans, 199
recommendations, 199
genetic effects, 197–198
background radiation, 198
basic concepts, 197
megamouse project, 198
mutations in Drosophila, 198
late effects of radiation, 192–196
concept of risk, 194–196
human experience, 192–193
hypotheses for late effects, 193–194
life-span shortening, 196
other late effects, 196
radiation hormesis, 194
types of late effects, 192
problems, 199–200
quantitative radiobiology, 184
microscopic autoradiography, 184
other methods, 184
survival curves, 184
radiation injury modifiers, 187–189
biological modifiers, 188
chemical modifiers, 187–188
dose fractionation, 189
overkill effect, 188
physical modifiers, 187
rationale, 171
study of radiobiology, 176–178
biological system, 177–178
general scheme, 176
sources of radiation, 176–177
survival curves, 184–186
definition, 184–185
equations, 185
shoulder, 185–186
theories of radiation injury, 179–182
indirect theory, 181–182
target theory, 180
tissue sensitivities, 186
cell populations, 186
cells, 186
law of Bergonie and Tribondeau, 186

types of damage, 186–187
potentially lethal damage, 187
sublethal damage, 186
types of exposure, 178–179
acute exposure, 178
chronic exposure, 179
experimental levels of exposure, 179
Radioimmunoassays (RIAs), 14, 83, 84
Radioiodine
therapy
hyperthyroidism, 117
imaging of metastases, 117
thyroid ablation, 117
volatile, 135
Radiological Society of North America (RSNA), 42
Radionuclide(s)
highly diffusible, 164
high-organ-uptake, 165
imaging procedures, 86
medical
half-lives of, 9
half-value layers of, 109
therapy, 112
dosimetry of, 160
radiation safety and, 98
radioiodine therapy, 117
release of patients, 119
room decontamination, 119
thyroid ablation, 118
Radiopharmaceuticals (RPs), 1, 68, 69
administration, 102
approval of new, 43
diagnostic, 81, 160
injection of, 139
internal doses from, 160
package inserts, 160
preparation, 104
radiation safety and, 95
remnants, 134
Radiopharmacy, 85, 87, 125
Radiotherapy, four Rs of, 189
Radiotoxicity, 133
Radium, discovery of, 2
Random errors, 70
RBE, *see* Relative biological effectiveness
RDD, *see* Radiation dispersion device
Recoil energy, 11
Regions of interest (ROIs), 68
Relative biological effectiveness (RBE), 34, 188
Relative error, 74, 75, 76
Relative standardization, 30
Reliability factor (RF), 76
Reportable events
EPA, 150
files, 150
incidents, 150
reports to individuals, 150
RES, *see* Reticuloendothelial system
Resolving time, 61
Respiration, definition of, 173
Respiratory chain, 174
Reticuloendothelial system (RES), 176
RF, *see* Reliability factor
RIAs, *see* Radioimmunoassays
Risk(s)
absolute, 195
comparison of, 195
concept of, 47
definition of, 194
malignancy, 195
Roentgen, William, 2, 41
ROIs, *see* Regions of interest
RPP, *see* Radiation protection program
RPs, *see* Radiopharmaceuticals
RSC, *see* Radiation safety committee
RSNA, *see* Radiological Society of North America
RSO, *see* Radiation safety officer
RSP, *see* Radiation safety program
Rutherford, Ernest, 2, 4

S

Safe handling of radioactivity, 103–122
laboratory rules, 112–113
minimizing external exposures, 103–110
effect of distance, 105–106
effect of shielding, 106–110
quantity of radioactivity used, 103–104
time of exposure, 104–105
other radionuclide therapies, 119–120
iodine-125, 120
iodine-131, 120
phosphorus-32, 119–120
strontium-89 chloride and ^{153}Sm-EDTMP, 120
yttrium-90, 120
preventing internal contamination, 110–112
accidental injection, 112
ingestion, 110
inhalation, 110–111
percutaneous absorption, 111–112
problems, 121
radiation hazards, 113–117
alpha emitters, 113
gamma emitters, 116
negatron emitters, 114–115

neutrons, 116–117
positron emitters, 115–116
radionuclide therapy, 117–119
radioiodine therapy, 117
release of patients, 119
room decontamination, 119
thyroid ablation, 118–119
rationale, 103
SCA, *see* Single-channel analyzer
Schilling test, 84
Scintillation
detectors, 59
applications, 67
Na(TI) detector, 65
principle, 66
single-channel analyzer, 66
SPECT, 67
window, 67
survey meter, 126
Shallow dose, 50
Single-channel analyzer (SCA), 59, 66, 67
Single-photon emission computerized tomography (SPECT), 57, 68, 81, 115
S.I. units, 38
SLD, *see* Sublethal damage
SNM, *see* Society of Nuclear Medicine
Snyder–Fisher phantom, 154
Society of Nuclear Medicine (SNM), 42, 45, 156
Solid wastes, 133, 134
Somatic cells, 174
Sommerfeld, Arnold, 3
Source, activity of, 9
Specific gamma constant, 37, 38
Specific ionization, 20, 34
Specific licenses, 48
SPECT, *see* Single-photon emission computerized tomography
Speed of light, 6
Spent reactor fuel (SRF), 132
SRF, *see* Spent reactor fuel
Standard error, 73
Standard man, 154, 155
Standard temperature and pressure (STP), 31
Statistical distributions
Gaussian distribution, 71
Poisson distribution, 70
Stochastic effects, 46, 49
STP, *see* Standard temperature and pressure
Strontium-89, 120
Sublethal damage (SLD), 186
Sublethal exposure, late effects in, 193
Surface monitors, 127
Survival curves
definition of, 184
low-LET, 186
mammalian cells, 185
Symbols, 205–210
Systematic errors, 70

T

Target theory, radiation injury, 179, 180
TC, *see* Time constant
Technetium-99m
decays, 17
imaging procedures, 85
Terrestrial radiation, 176
Thallium-201 decays, 15
Theory of relativity, Einstein's, 3
Thermoluminescent dosimeter (TLD) badges, 32, 50, 59, 141
Thin-layer chromatography (TLC), 103
Third circulation, 176
Thomson, J.J., 2
Threshold linear hypothesis (TLH), 194
Thyroid ablation, 117, 118
TI, *see* Transportation index
Time, 6
Time constant (TC), 62
Tissue
sensitivities
cell populations, 186
cells, 186
law of Bergonie and Tribondeau, 186
weighting factors, 34
TLC, *see* Thin-layer chromatography
TLD badges, *see* Thermoluminescent dosimeter badges
TLH, *see* Threshold linear hypothesis
Total counts collected, 73
Transportation index (TI), 44
Transuranic wastes (TRU), 132
TRU, *see* Transuranic wastes

U

Uncertainty, principle of, 4
United Nations Food and Agricultural Organization (FAO), 43
United Nations Scientific Committee on the Effects of Atomic Radiation (UNSCEAR), 43
Units, interconversion of, 211
Units of radiation exposure and dose, 29–40
basic concepts, 29–34
absorbed dose, 32
activity, 30–31

effective dose, 33–34
equivalent dose, 32–33
exposure, 31–32
relative biological effectiveness, 34
other concepts, 34–35
f value, 35
linear energy transfer, 35
range of beta particles, 35
specific ionization, 34
W value, 35
problems, 39
rationale, 29
S.I. units, 38–39
specific gamma constant, 37–38
UNSCEAR, *see* United Nations Scientific Committee on the Effects of Atomic Radiation
U.S. Centers for Disease Control (CDC), 43

V

Viruses, 172
Volatile radioiodine, 135

W

Warm areas, 83
Waste(s)
disposal, *see* Radiation surveys and waste disposal
high-level, 132
liquid, 133, 135
low-level, 133
management, 134
nuclear medicine, 133
solid, 133, 134
transportation of, 136
transuranic, 132
Water, properties of, 24
WHO, *see* World Health Organization
Whole-body exposure, 139, 189, 190
Wipe-test counters
design, 63
positive wipes, 63
Wipe-test monitoring, 125, 129
Wipe-test survey record, 129
World Health Organization (WHO), 43
W value, 35

X

x-rays, 2, 41

Y

Yttrium-90, 120